The Scientific Basis of Oral Health Education

ISBN 0 904588 84X

Printed and bound by
Dennis Barber Limited,
Lowestoft, Suffolk

The Scientific Basis of Oral Health Education

R S Levine OBE
General Dental Practitioner and Independent Scientific Adviser
370 Alwoodley Lane
Leeds
LS17 7DN

C R Stillman-Lowe
Independent Oral Health Promotion Adviser
7 Broadwater Road
Twyford
Reading
RG10 0EX

2004

Published by the British Dental Association
64 Wimpole Street, London, W1G 8YS

Preface

The first edition of *The Scientific Basis of Dental Health Education* appeared in 1976 and was a slim booklet with a green cover. It arose from a joint attempt by the British Association for the Study of Community Dentistry and the Health Education Council, who published it, to refine and standardize the advice given to the public and to ensure that such advice was scientifically sound. The need for this document grew from the problem of confusing and sometimes conflicting dental health education messages being provided by professional and commercial bodies. The strength of the original document was that it came from an independent and authoritative source and was based on a consensus of scientific opinion from a group of the leading dental experts of the day.

Over the intervening quarter century, the document grew through four editions to become one of the most widely used and accepted sources of information on dental health, both in the UK and abroad. Now, the emergence of a more formalized system of evidence-based clinical practice, together with an increased emphasis on evidence-based oral health promotion, has made it essential to completely recast it for the 21st century. This book introduces a simple system for indicating the level of scientific evidence supporting a series of key statements on oral health. Following consultation with government and a range of professional bodies, both the format and the style have been changed to increase its readability and value to a wider range of user groups. New topics have been included in response to requests and the changing pattern of oral health. There is also a new series of appendices. These include information on smoking cessation, general healthy eating and sensible drinking guidelines, the eruption dates of teeth, first aid for traumatized teeth and evidence-based dentistry websites, for those who wish to keep up-to-date with new developments. In keeping with the wider range of oral topics now included, the title of this new edition has been changed to *The Scientific Basis of Oral Health Education*. To keep the book within a reasonable length, however, it does not attempt to cover the full scope of oral health promotion: this is covered well by other textbooks, listed in the further reading section.

As before, it is hoped that this new edition will be used by dental schools dental postgraduate deans and directors to help standardize undergraduate and postgraduate teaching and by professionals complementary to dentistry, whose role within the dental team has developed significantly since 1976. Those involved in general healthcare, such as medical practitioners, school nurses, health visitors, midwives, dieticians and pharmacists also have a vital role to play in oral health promotion, and it is hoped that this publication will be of value to them. Oral health promotion staff in the Community Dental Service frequently provide training for people who can influence health in the wider community, such as teachers, child carers and peer educators, and they can safely rely on the messages in this book as the basis for their programmes. Finally, it must be recognized that oral health education material is provided by a wide range of agencies, including government and professional bodies, charities, and commercial organizations in the form of both patient education material and for product promotion, much of which is of the highest standard. This too should conform to agreed expert opinion and it is hoped that this publication will be of assistance to these bodies.

Above all, this document is offered in the sincere belief that oral health education is one of our most important responsibilities and must be approached with the same dedication and professional quality standards that are applied to the operative treatment of disease. Only by offering the public consistent and soundly based advice can we hope that health education messages achieve their intended function of enabling individuals to control and improve their own health, as part of a comprehensive programme of national and local public health initiatives designed to tackle the determinants of poor health.

Ronnie Levine and Catherine Stillman-Lowe
May 2004

v

Acknowledgements

With the closure of the Health Education Authority in 2000, the future of *The Scientific Basis of Dental Health Education* was thrown into doubt. We are grateful to the Health Development Agency and the Dental Practice Board for commissioning and publishing a revised fourth edition of the document in 2001. The support of many professionals for a fifth edition, more widely available, was substantial, and to those who put the case forcefully to us, including the then Chair of the National Oral Health Promotion Group and the President of the British Dental Hygienists' Association, we are also indebted.

As with the previous editions, a considerable debt of gratitude is owed to the panel of expert advisers, including a number of new members as well as several who were involved in the earlier editions. They have been generous with their time and advice to help ensure that the document remains a consensus of expert opinion. For the first time, with this edition, a formal consultation process with a wide range of professional bodies and agencies has taken place to help shape and develop the book. We are grateful to all those who took the time and contributed to this, so that the book could reflect the needs of the whole dental team.

A guide to using this book

The aim of this book is to provide a sound basis for giving information and advice on the main aspects of oral health. The summary that follows gives a brief overview of the main oral diseases and some other oral conditions, together with four key messages. These key messages are a consensus of expert opinion and should form the basis of all oral health advice given to the public.

Chapters 1 to 11 cover the various diseases that can affect the teeth and mouth as a whole together with information on their causes and means of prevention, including advice for the under fives and older people.

Throughout this document, important statements are given at the end of each chapter in the form of key points. In order to indicate the level of supporting scientific evidence for each of these key points a simple scheme called Evidence Base is used:

- Evidence Base A: Statements supported by very strong evidence from pooled research data (meta-analysis) or systematic literature reviews.

- Evidence Base B: Statements supported by the majority of relevant research studies.

- Evidence Base C: Statements that cannot be supported by a substantial body of research evidence, but where there is a consensus of scientific and professional opinion to support the statement.

More detailed information on Evidence Base is given in Chapter 12, together with sections on health education and the nature of scientific evidence.

Summary

The two most common oral diseases are tooth decay, or dental caries and gum disease, properly known as *periodontal disease*. The principal cause of dental caries is the frequent consumption of sugars, mainly in confectionery, snack foods and soft drinks, acting on the layer of bacteria on the tooth surface, which we call plaque. The sugars are rapidly converted into acid by plaque bacteria and the build up of acid attacks the tooth surface causing a cavity and if untreated, destruction of the tooth with pain and possibly infection.

The common form of periodontal disease is caused by poor oral hygiene allowing bacteria in the form of plaque to build up round the necks of the teeth. The toxins released from plaque cause inflammation of the gums, a condition known as gingivitis. The later stage of periodontitis develops when the supporting bone around the teeth becomes progressively destroyed, so that the teeth become loose and painful. Smoking is now recognized as a related cause. Unlike tooth decay, which is usually a rapid process, periodontal disease can take many years to reach the stage where teeth become loose and may be lost. In the UK the annual cost to the National Health Service for the treatment of these two conditions now exceeds £2 billion.

Dental erosion appears to be an increasing problem, which causes wearing away of the surface of the teeth. The cause is usually acid in the soft drinks and juices increasingly being consumed by children and young adults, 50% of whom are now affected to some degree. Erosion can also be caused by gastric regurgitation, as can occur in pregnancy, or due to conditions such as hiatus hernia or bulimia.

There are many other diseases that occur in the mouth and there are some conditions arising elsewhere in the body that can have a visible effect within the mouth, such as pregnancy, anaemia and HIV infection (AIDS). The most life-threatening oral disease is oral cancer. This condition is nearly as common as cervical cancer in the UK, with about 4,500 new cases each year, most being smoking or alcohol related. About half of these cases prove fatal, but early diagnosis greatly improves the chance of survival. Dental patients who wish to give up smoking should be offered appropriate support to do so.

Dental disease is not an inevitable part of life and research has shown that much can be prevented by changes in behaviour. Such changes require the knowledge and skills to make healthy choices and these in turn are influenced by social and economic pressures, both on individuals and communities. These factors may account for the persistence of high levels of dental caries in economically depressed communities.

To promote good oral health there are four key messages:

1. Diet: reduce the consumption and especially the frequency of intake of drinks, confectionery and foods with sugars.
The consumption of sugars, both the frequency and the amount, is important in determining the rate of tooth decay. When sugars are consumed, they should be part of a meal rather than between meals. Snacks and drinks should be free of added sugars, whenever possible. The frequent consumption of acidic drinks (such as fruit juice, squashes or carbonated drinks) should be avoided to help prevent dental erosion.

2. Toothbrushing: clean the teeth thoroughly twice every day with a fluoride toothpaste.
Effective daily toothbrushing with a fluoride toothpaste is the best way of preventing both caries and periodontal disease. Other oral hygiene aids such as floss and interdental brushes are best used after they have been demonstrated by a dentist, therapist or hygienist. Thorough brushing of all tooth surfaces and gum margins twice every day is of more value than more frequent cursory brushing, and a gentle scrub technique should be advised. A small soft-to-medium texture toothbrush should be used to allow all tooth surfaces and gum margins to be cleaned easily and comfortably. Effective toothbrushing with a fluoride toothpaste will help control caries provided that the diet is also favourable.

3. Fluoride: fluoridation of the water supply is a safe and highly effective public health measure.
Water fluoridation should be targeted at communities with higher caries levels. Where it is not technically feasible other fluoride strategies should be employed, such as programmes to promote the use of fluoride toothpaste.

4. Dental attendance: have an oral examination every year.
Everyone, irrespective of age and dental condition, should have an oral examination approximately once a year so that cases of oral cancer or other oral diseases can be detected early and treated. This advice also applies to those without any natural teeth. Children and those at risk from oral disease, including smokers, may need to be seen more frequently, as advised by the dentist.

Contents

Dental caries

Who gets caries?

This condition is often said to be the most common affecting mankind. This was true for much of the western developed world during the last century, but not for Asia and Africa. Within Europe and North America, the level of caries appeared to reach a peak in the 1960s and has decreased in prevalence during the last 30 years. Nevertheless it remains a major health problem for people of all ages. Its peak activity occurs during childhood. In the UK, national surveys are undertaken at regular intervals by the British Association for the Study of Community Dentistry. The 2001/2 national survey found at least one decayed tooth in 39% of five-year-olds in England, 53% in Wales, and 55% in Scotland. The mean number of decayed teeth per child being, 1.47, 2.26 and 2.55 respectively.[1] In Northern Ireland in 1997/8, over 60% of five-year-olds had caries experience, and the average number of decayed teeth per child was 2.9.[2]

There are wide variations in caries prevalence, often within small geographical areas and this is related to two social factors. Firstly, like many other diseases, it has become apparent that dental caries is essentially a disease associated with social deprivation. In the UK, low levels of caries can now be seen in the more affluent areas, especially in southern England. However, levels remain high in children in many inner city socially deprived areas of Wales, Scotland and Northern Ireland, and northern parts of England. The second factor is ethnicity and is a complex one, possibly related to different dietary and toothbrushing practices within different cultures. Some children of Asian ethnic background, including children of non-English speaking mothers, have the highest caries rates for deciduous teeth. One study of five-year olds found that Asian children had 60% more decayed teeth than white children living in the same towns.[3] However, this difference is not apparent in the permanent teeth of older children.

How caries affects teeth

Dental caries affects the tooth itself. The consequences of caries are familiar to most people (Fig. 1.1).

The process begins at the tooth surface but is often hidden from sight in the fissures (grooves) or between the teeth. Where it is visible the initial appearance may be as a chalky white patch or ring around the neck of the tooth or as a shadow or staining on the biting surface (Fig. 1.2).

The chalky appearance is due to the enamel surface having lost some of the calcium and phosphate mineral crystals of which it is largely composed. This

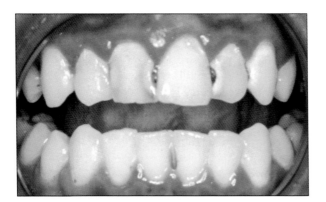

Fig. 1.1 Dental caries.

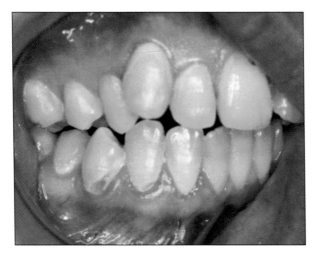

Fig. 1.2 Caries at the necks of teeth, from 'white spot' stage to cavitation.

process is called *demineralization*. The destructive process can then spread into the dentine (the softer, sensitive part of the tooth beneath the enamel). The weakened enamel then collapses to form a cavity and the tooth is progressively destroyed. Caries causes progressive destruction of the crowns of the teeth often accompanied by severe pain and infection. The roots of teeth can also be attacked should they become exposed by gum recession and this is more common in older adults.

Cause

The basic process that causes caries is sometimes called an 'acid attack'.

Caries begins within the plaque on the tooth surface following the consumption of sugars in drinks and foods.

- When sugars enter the mouth they are rapidly absorbed by the bacteria in the plaque layer on the surfaces of the teeth.

- Inside the bacterial cells the sugars are converted by metabolic processes into organic acids as a waste product and excreted into the plaque fluid.

- The acids accumulate in the plaque layer and cause demineralization of the enamel surface.

SUGARS —> PLAQUE —> ACID —> DEMINERALIZATION

This 'acid attack' is more accurately described as a 'demineralization episode' caused by the action of plaque bacteria on sugars entering the mouth.

Sucrose and glucose are the most important dietary sugars as they are added to many food products and beverages during manufacture. As table sugar, sucrose is often added during cooking or immediately before consumption. These simple sugars can enter the plaque bacteria and be metabolized within minutes of being consumed. Since plaque covers most tooth surfaces and reforms quickly after brushing, when acid forms within the plaque it acts almost like a layer of acid-soaked blotting paper on the teeth.

Most people will consume some sugars as part of the everyday diet, but not everyone develops caries. To explain why this is so we must look in more detail at the factors that determine the risk from decay.

The pattern and severity of attack are determined by two groups of factors – those factors that influence the tooth's resistance to attack and those, in the environment of the tooth, which influence the severity of the attack.

The tooth's resistance

Largely because of their shape or position in the mouth some teeth are more resistant to attack than others. For example, in young people lower front teeth rarely decay because they don't have any grooves or fissures in which plaque can stagnate and they are bathed by saliva, which is beneficial. In contrast, the first permanent molar teeth have the highest decay rate because the deep fissures on the biting surfaces are difficult to clean.

In the UK, neither malnutrition in the mother during pregnancy, nor in the child after birth, is likely to have any appreciable effect on the susceptibility of the teeth to decay. Calcium cannot be removed from the mother's teeth by the foetus during pregnancy or during lactation. The one factor that has been shown beyond doubt to reduce the rate of decay is fluoride and this is described below and in Chapter 2.

The tooth's environment

The important factors within the mouth that interact to influence the severity of attack are plaque, dietary sugars, saliva and fluoride.

Sugars from the diet pass into the plaque within seconds of consumption. Many plaque bacteria use sugars as their source of energy and rapidly produce acid as a by-product. As acid is generated, it accumulates in the plaque layer and acidity in the plaque increases. Acidity is measured on the *pH* scale, and the lower the figure, the greater the degree of acidity. Figure 1.3 shows the effect of a sugar intake on plaque pH. The fall in plaque pH when sugars enter the mouth and the subsequent recovery as shown in the diagram is called the 'Stephan curve'. This demineralization-remineralization episode is sometimes referred to as an 'acid attack'.

Within minutes of a sugar intake, sufficient acid may be generated within the absorbent plaque layer to cause a small outflow of calcium and phosphate from the enamel resulting in a tiny degree of demineralization. After a period of time (usually about 20 minutes, but possibly up to two hours), the acid will have dissipated and the lost mineral may be slowly replaced from the saliva. This

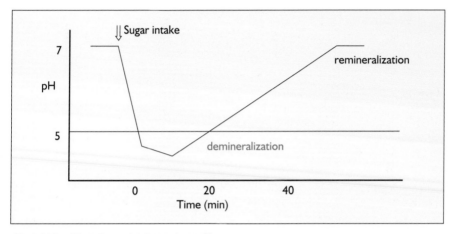

Fig. 1.3 The effect of sugar intake on plaque pH.

process is called remineralization. However, if sugars are consumed frequently during the day, especially without the presence of other food or liquids that might dilute or help neutralize the acid, then the amount of demineralization may outweigh remineralization. This situation is illustrated in Figure 1.4a where a frequent intake of sugars during the day leads to an unfavourable proportion of total demineralization to remineralization periods, while an infrequent sugars intake results in a more favourable proportion as seen in Figure 1.4b.

If this imbalance persists over a period of time, then the gradual loss of mineral from the enamel may lead to its eventual breakdown and the formation of a cavity.

The type of bacteria that predominate within the plaque is influenced by the diet. Frequent consumption of sugars has been shown to encourage the multiplication of bacteria that use sugars and can efficiently convert them to acid and it also increases the thickness of the plaque layer. The most commonly implicated plaque organism is *Strepococcus mutans*, however there are many other types that metabolize sugars to form acid. The proportion of these decay-causing bacteria falls when the amount and frequency of dietary sugars are reduced.

However, the mouth has its own defence mechanisms. While these are not fully understood, saliva is clearly the most important as it bathes the plaque on the tooth surface and helps to neutralize the acids and wash away sugars. This

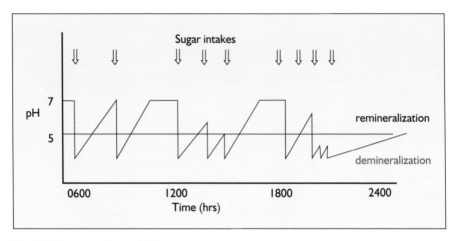

Fig. 1.4a Frequency of sugars intake.

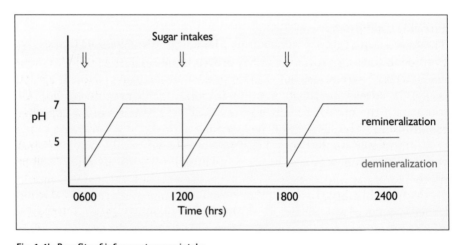

Fig. 1.4b Benefits of infrequent sugars intake.

effect is enhanced if salivary flow after sugary snacks is stimulated for example by vegetables, cheese or sugar-free chewing gum. In addition, at the very earliest stages of the decay process, the tooth surface may 'heal' or 'remineralize' by deposition from saliva of calcium and phosphate, together with fluoride, which accelerates the healing process.

6

The early decay process may be seen as a contest fought at the tooth surface between the acids (resulting from the intake of sugars) causing demineralization of the tooth surface and a number of factors including fluoride and saliva promoting the remineralization of the tooth surface.

Prevention

There are two ways for individuals to reduce the risk of caries. The first is by using fluoride, easily and effectively done by brushing twice-daily with a fluoride toothpaste. The second is to reduce the severity of attack by decreasing the frequency and amount of consumption of sugars, the two being strongly linked. These methods will be discussed separately, but should be used together in order to improve or maintain oral health.

Fluoride

Fluoride toothpaste
The daily use of a fluoride toothpaste is a highly effective method of delivering fluoride to the tooth surface and has proved to be a major benefit. To some extent its use has removed the need for professionally applied fluoride agents, except in special circumstances. To increase the benefit from fluoride toothpaste, the mouth should not be rinsed with water from a cup after toothbrushing. The paste should be spat out and the mouth rinsed with a little water transferred on the brush if desired. Care should be taken to ensure that young children do not eat toothpaste and brushing should be supervised by parents for those under seven years of age. It is advised that parents should finish off the brushing to ensure that it has been done effectively and that the biting surfaces of any newly erupted teeth are cleaned, as they can be easily missed. The use of only a small pea-sized amount of toothpaste (with just a tiny smear for babies) is recommended by both the dental profession and manufacturers for children under seven years of age.[4] When fluoride drops or tablets are used, they should be given at a different time of day to brushing.

Water fluoridation
There are many natural sources of dietary fluoride, such as fish (bones) and tea and the drinking water supply in some areas. However, the most effective, safe and efficient public health measure for reducing dental caries is the

fluoridation of public drinking water at a level of one part of fluoride per one million parts of water (1 ppm), which is equivalent to 1 mg F/litre. This is regarded as an optimum level. Since caries levels have fallen in many parts of the UK in the last 20 years, most experts now believe that water fluoridation should be targeted at areas where decay levels remain high.

Other fluoride agents

For extra protection against caries, fluoride gels and varnishes are effective and can be applied to the teeth by dentists, therapists and hygienists. For maximum benefit these should be applied every three or four months. Fluoride mouthrinses are also effective and are available for home use. These agents are of greatest value for the individuals who are most at risk to caries (see page 1).

Fluoride tablets and drops

Fluoride drops and tablets are available on prescription from dentists and doctors in the UK and may be purchased from pharmacists without a prescription. They were originally introduced to mimic the effect of water fluoridation by raising the dietary fluoride intake to what was considered to be an optimal level for caries control. For maximum effectiveness, daily administration from infancy until adolescence was required, although compliance with this regime was recognized as a frequent problem. Over the years the recommended dosage schedule has been reduced because of concerns that their use may be associated with a higher incidence of enamel fluorosis (see page 16). While initially seen as a potential public health measure, the introduction of fluoride toothpaste into the UK in the early 1970s has proved to be far more effective. Some experts now doubt the extent of any additional benefit that their use may provide beyond that achieved by effective twice-daily toothbrushing with a fluoride toothpaste. Today, their use should be confined to those at very high risk to caries or to those for whom dental treatment may be complicated by their general health (see page 14). Because of compliance problems, some clinicians prefer to rely on professionally applied topical fluoride agents such as fluoride varnishes or gels where additional measures are required. Fluoride drops or tablets should not be given in areas that have the optimum level of fluoride in the water supply and parents should therefore seek professional advice before use.

More information on fluoride is given in Chapter 2.

Diet

Sugars in our diet

Food industry statistics estimate that almost half of the sucrose consumed by the public is sold as packaged sugar and about half is used by food, drink and confectionery manufacturers. The major industrial use of sucrose is the production of confectionery, which accounts for about a quarter of the total used in manufacturing, while the soft drinks industry uses about one fifth.

Nearly three-quarters of all sugars in the UK diet are added to foods during manufacture, cooking or before consumption. Confectionery, soft drinks, cakes, biscuits and table sugar (in tea and coffee, for example) are often consumed between meals and their frequent consumption is strongly linked to decay. The other sugars in the diet are naturally present in foods such as whole fruit, vegetables and milk. When sugars are consumed as part of these foods they are considered to be relatively unimportant as a cause of decay.

Dietary advice

Dietary advice should be aimed at changing the pattern of consumption of sugars with the aim of reducing the frequency and amount of consumption. The elimination of one or two sugar-sweetened items each day may be sufficient to enable remineralization of the teeth to prevail over demineralization, especially if fluoride from water or toothpaste is available. Food and drinks containing added sugars should be identified and limited, especially between meals. While fresh fruit and vegetables naturally contain sugars, their consumption is not linked to decay and they have an important place in our diet. Fruit juice and dried fruit can adversely affect teeth because of their high concentration of sugars and are not recommended for consumption between meals. Concentrated fruit juices should be well diluted with water. However, plain water is the safest drink as far as the teeth are concerned.

Parents and carers of infants should be warned of the dangers of putting fruit juice or sugars-sweetened drinks into feeding bottles, valve-type and reservoir feeders for the child to hold, especially in bed. Such practices result in almost continuous bathing of the enamel with sugars and lead to rapid tooth destruction. From six months of age, infants should be introduced to drinking from a cup. Free-flowing lidded feeding cups can help avoid spills in the early stages, before infants move on to an open beaker or cup. Feeding bottles should be discouraged after the age of 12 months.

People should also be encouraged to study the nutritional labels of food and drinks, and avoid frequently consuming those with high levels of sugars. The Food Standards Agency suggests a figure of 2g of sugars per 100g as a low sugar content and 10g per 100g as a high content. Foods and drinks may contain added sugars other than sucrose. Glucose, maltose and fructose (when listed as an added sugar) are as likely to cause decay as sucrose and should not be used in infant health drinks and foods unless they are consumed only at mealtimes.

The use of sugars in medicines should also be strongly discouraged and sugar-free liquid medicines should be chosen by prescribers and when buying non-prescription medicines, whenever possible. If children have a long-term medical condition, parents and carers should request clinicians to prescribe sugar-free liquid medicines or preferably, tablets instead of liquids.

Preferable snacks and drinks for between-meal consumption

For between-meal snacks and drinks, raw vegetables such as carrots, fresh fruit, bread, low-fat unsweetened yoghurt, lower-fat cheese, skimmed or semi-skimmed milk and water can be recommended. Whole cow's milk should only be used as a main milk drink after the age of one year. Children between one and two years of age need whole milk. Between the ages of two and five years, provided they are eating a good varied diet, semi-skimmed milk can be introduced. Skimmed milk should not be given before the age of five. Milk and water are the only safe drinks for the teeth.

More information on diet and caries can be found in Chapter 3.

Plaque control

Caries cannot develop without the presence of plaque, which is needed to convert dietary sugars into acid. Some research studies have shown that highly efficient toothbrushing techniques can reduce caries. But, plaque removal by normal toothbrushing alone does not appear to be as effective. Some plaque is left in fissures and other stagnation sites where caries occurs and plaque rapidly reforms on cleaned tooth surfaces. However brushing with a fluoride toothpaste combines plaque removal with the application of fluoride to the tooth surface and has proved to be highly effective.

Eating crisp or crunchy foods such as apples or raw carrots will not remove plaque effectively. However they are suitable snack foods and are an important part of a healthy diet.

More information on plaque control can be found in Chapter 5.

Fissure sealants

A further way of helping to prevent dental caries is for a plastic film to be professionally applied to the pits and fissures of teeth as soon as possible after the teeth grow into the mouth. For the permanent molar teeth this is from the age of six years. The sealant prevents access of plaque and plaque acids to the enamel surface. Clinical trials have shown that sealants can be well retained and prevent caries. However, they are only effective on the biting surfaces of teeth. They are more cost effective in children at higher risk to caries and should be considered when there is a risk to general health from caries or dental treatment. In all cases fissure sealants should be seen as one part of a comprehensive preventive plan.

Key points
- Caries is caused by the action of sugars on the bacterial plaque covering the teeth. *Evidence Base A*

- Caries occurs when demineralization of the tooth surface exceeds remineralization. *Evidence Base A*

- The risk of developing caries can be reduced by avoiding sugars between meals and at bedtime. *Evidence Base B*

- The risk of developing caries can be reduced by brushing with a fluoride toothpaste twice daily. *Evidence Base A*

- Never leave infants with sugars-sweetened drinks in feeding bottles or cups, especially at bedtime. *Evidence Base B*

- Caries occurs in all populations and age groups but is more common amongst children and disadvantaged groups. *Evidence Base A*

2 Fluoride

Fluoride toothpaste

Fluoride toothpaste, which came into general use in the UK in the early 1970s, is now recognized as a development of the greatest importance to dental health. It is the most cost-effective topical fluoride agent for personal use and is thought to be the main reason for the decline in caries prevalence in Europe during the last 30 years. Fluoride toothpastes are currently available in three concentration ranges:

- Lower fluoride pastes containing less than 600 ppm;
- Standard pastes containing about 1000–1500 ppm;
- High concentration pastes containing over 2000 ppm.

The lower fluoride formulations were introduced to meet the concern that young children might ingest excessive fluoride. However, research has shown that the effectiveness of fluoride toothpastes increases with the fluoride concentration and there is no clear evidence that pastes containing less than 1000 ppm are effective. The use of lower concentration pastes may only be justified for children who are at low risk to caries, living in a fluoridated area or receiving fluoride supplements. Indicators of low risk include little evidence of past caries activity and good oral hygiene suggesting regular use of fluoride toothpaste. Toothpastes containing 1000 to 1500 ppm are highly effective and should be used by all children from seven years of age. Some toothpastes marketed as 'children's toothpaste' contain 1000 ppm but have a milder flavouring to provide a more acceptable taste for children. The labeling of toothpastes remains unsatisfactory as the total fluoride content is not clearly marked in a simple form for the public to recognize.

While brands with similar fluoride concentrations may be equally effective, other components of the formulation may influence overall benefit. A number of leading brands have been independently evaluated in published long-term clinical trials in order to ensure efficacy. There is evidence that rinsing with water immediately after brushing with fluoride toothpaste reduces the benefit both in relation to the development of new cavities and the prevention of recurrent caries around fillings. It is preferable simply to spit out the paste and, if desired, the mouth rinsed with a little water transferred on the brush.

Fluoridation

Fluorides are compounds of the chemical element fluorine. They are widely found in nature, in some foods such as fish (bones), in some plants such as tea, in beer and in some natural water supplies. The link between the presence of fluoride in public water supplies and reduced caries experience was first noticed early last century and has now been demonstrated by over 130 surveys in more than 20 countries including the UK. These surveys confirm that fluoride in the water at a concentration of about one part per million (1 ppm) reduces caries levels by up to half compared to similar non-fluoride areas. In 1945, Grand Rapids in the USA became the first community to have its water supply artificially adjusted to contain 1 ppm fluoride. Since then many cities around the world have followed, the largest schemes in the UK being in Birmingham, including parts of the West Midlands and Newcastle upon Tyne, where the improvement in children's dental health has been dramatic since fluoridation began.

The safety of water fluoridation is well documented. Numerous studies in both natural and artificially fluoridated areas have failed to show any adverse effect on general health at the level of 1 ppm, though fluoridation may be associated with an increase in dental fluorosis. One of the most authoritative reports is that of the Royal College of Physicians of England (1976). Fluoride's effectiveness and safety were upheld in the Court of Session judgment in Edinburgh in 1983.

Analysis of the reduction in treatment need after fluoridation has shown savings in manpower and resources. A large fall in the numbers of extractions and general anaesthetics administered to children has been reported. Furthermore, there is evidence from Scotland that the discontinuation of water fluoridation can result in a return to higher caries levels, despite the benefit of fluoride toothpaste. A 25% increase in caries prevalence was recorded five years after parts of Scotland were de-fluoridated. However, in some countries no change in caries levels has been seen after de-fluoridation. This might be due to changes in diet or the increased use of fluoride toothpaste.

The evidence for the safety and benefits of fluoridation has led to support

13

from the Committee on Child Health Services (1976), the Royal Commission of Inquiry into the Health Service (1979), the 1981 report of the Dental Strategy Review Group, The World Health Organization (1998), the Independent Inquiry into Inequalities in Health (1998), the Medical Research Council (2002) and the All Party Parliamentary Primary Care & Public Health Group (2003). This opinion has been embodied in guidance documents from the Department of Health, including *An Oral Health Strategy for England* (1994), *Modernising NHS Dentistry – Implementing the NHS Plan* (2000) and in England and Wales, the Water Act 2004.

A recent authoritative systematic review of 214 water fluoridation studies by the University of York found no clear evidence for a detrimental effect on general health.[5] The review concluded that the best available evidence suggests that fluoridation of the drinking water supply does reduce caries prevalence. However, it did conclude that the quality of many studies, which were done decades ago, did not meet today's rigorous research standards and that further research was needed to improve the evidence base on the safety and efficacy of water fluoridation.

While in some areas falling caries prevalence has reduced the absolute benefit to be gained from water fluoridation, in communities where prevalence remains high, often because of social and economic factors, there are significant potential benefits. Because of these changes, the consensus of expert opinion is that water fluoridation should be targeted at areas with higher caries levels.

Fluoride tablets and drops

Supplementing the diet of children during the period of tooth development with fluoride in the form of tablets and drops is no longer considered to be an effective public health measure. Twice-daily toothbrushing with a fluoride toothpaste has proved to be highly effective and some experts believe that any additional benefit from the use of fluoride supplements may be small. Over the years the recommended dosage schedule has been reduced because of concerns that their use may be associated with a higher incidence of enamel fluorosis (see page 16).

Fluoride dietary supplements may be considered for those for whom the consequences of decay pose a hazard to general health or for whom dental treatment would be difficult because of their medical or physical condition. These groups include children with heart disease or cardiac defects who need

14

pre-operative antibiotic cover for any dental procedure, as well as children prone to infection because of systemic disorders. Special needs children, those with mental or physical disabilities, may be more at risk to dental disease because of oral hygiene and dietary problems and may find dental treatment, when needed, difficult or frightening. All of these children could benefit from fluoride supplements. The need for their use should be determined with dental advice and reviewed at intervals. Parents and carers should be advised of the benefits, and risks and especially of the long-term commitment, to the use of this measure, and of the importance of safe storage away from the reach of children.

The main problem with the use of fluoride dietary supplements is compliance with the required daily regime over the whole period of tooth formation. A stop-start pattern of use is unlikely to provide significant benefit. Some experts believe that compliance is likely to be higher in motivated families where the children may have a low risk of developing caries, while conversely, compliance may be poor in areas of social deprivation where the caries risk and the need for preventive measures is greater.

Fluoride supplements are licensed products and dosages appear in the *British National Formulary/Dental Practitioners' Formulary* as follows.

Daily dosage schedule for areas with less than 0.3 ppm F in the water supply:

- 6 months to 3 years – 0.25 mg F (0.5 mg NaF)

- 3 years up to 6 years – 0.5 mg F (1.1 mg NaF)

- 6 years and over – 1.0 mg F (2.2 mg NaF)

Once started, the continued need for fluoride supplements should be reviewed at intervals. It is generally advised that for maximum benefit their use be continued until the appearance of the second molar teeth, usually at about 11 to 12 years of age. However, this advice is based on the pre-eruptive effect of the ingested fluoride. Some experts believe that by allowing the tablets to dissolve slowly in the mouth a more beneficial topical post-eruptive effect may be achieved, both for older children and adults who may be at risk to caries.

For areas with 0.3 ppm or more F in the water supply a lower dosage should be considered. While the schedule is provided for guidance, different dosages may be appropriate for individual patients and recommended dosages are periodically reviewed by expert groups.

In prescribing for individual patients, practitioners should determine the appropriate dosage schedule based on benefit, risk and compliance considerations and both the need and dosage should be reviewed at intervals. Fluoride supplements should be given daily, but the dose must not be increased if days are missed. No supplements should be given in areas where the water supply contains more than 0.7 ppm F. Local water companies and the Community Dental Service can confirm the fluoride content of the water supply.

Fluoridated milk

The use of fluoridated milk for dental caries prevention was first proposed in the 1950s and school-based fluoridated milk programmes are now operating in 15 countries ranging from Russia to Chile. In the UK, over 17,000 children in over 200 schools drink fluoridated milk at school as part of a programme that began in 1993 and was coordinated by the Liverpool Dental School. An additional potential benefit is that fluoridated milk may help displace sweetened soft drinks from the refrigerated vending machines found in many schools.

Results from early clinical trials indicate a reduction in caries levels comparable to those achieved by water fluoridation. However the organization and maintenance of school-based programmes can pose problems where there is high absenteeism in infant and primary schools, or difficulty with the reliability of the milk distribution process.

Enamel fluorosis

This much publicized condition presents as opaque or white areas, lines or flecks in the enamel surface and are most noticeable when they occur on front teeth. While these opacities can be due to a number of causes, one is the ingestion of excessive fluoride during the period of enamel formation. For incisor teeth the period of greatest risk is between 15 and 30 months of age. The more severe, cosmetically unacceptable forms are uncommon in the UK, but may result from the use of fluoride dietary supplements in optimally fluoridated areas or from the eating of fluoride toothpaste in early childhood. The use of fluoride toothpaste in areas with optimally fluoridated water supplies has been shown by surveys using sensitive photographic recording to result in only a small increase in the mildest forms, which mostly pass unnoticed. No increase in moderate or severe forms has yet been detected, and simple techniques are available to improve the appearance of affected teeth. Nevertheless, this is an area of concern to both the public and the dental professions and care should be taken to ensure that young children do not ingest excessive amounts of fluoride toothpaste, especially in fluoridated areas or when fluoride supplements are used. While manufacturers rightly endeavour to make the taste of children's toothpaste attractive, there is concern that the use of food flavouring such as strawberry may encourage excessive consumption.

To reduce the risk of fluorosis, parents should supervise toothbrushing of children under seven years of age and should place an amount of toothpaste no greater than the size of a small pea on the brush (or a small smear for babies). Brushing should be done normally no more than twice each day and the child should be encouraged to spit out afterwards, rather than rinse with water. Supervision will continue to be beneficial beyond this age. When fluoride drops or tablets are used, they should be given at a different time of day to brushing.

How does fluoride work?

Teeth and bone are composed largely of a crystalline mineral compound of calcium and phosphate called *hydroxyapatite*. Research over the past 60 years has shown that fluoride produces its effect in a number of different ways which combine to slow and help prevent the decay process and also to reverse decay in its early stages. These are given below in the order of effectiveness.

- *Enhanced remineralization* – Very low levels of fluoride in the plaque and saliva are able to alter the chemical balance between demineralization of the enamel and remineralization. The effect favours the remineralisation process, allowing the early carious attack on enamel to be reversed and new mineral crystals, with better structure and greater acid resistance, to be deposited. This is the mechanism by which fluoride toothpaste is thought to work and appears to be the most important.

- *Reduced acid production* – Fluoride is concentrated in the plaque layer on the surfaces of the teeth and reduces the conversion of dietary sugars into acid by plaque bacteria. Fluoride toothpaste also invokes this mechanism.

- *Fluoride substitution* – Fluoride entering the developing teeth from the

17

diet via the blood stream is incorporated into the new mineral crystals. The partly fluoridated hydroxyapatite that is formed is theoretically more resistant to acid attack than that formed without fluoride.

- *Reduced pit and fissure depth* – The parts of the teeth most susceptible to caries are the natural pits and grooves, or fissures on the biting surfaces of back teeth. Fluoride entering the developing teeth at an early stage appears to result in reduced pit and fissure depth.

The use of fluoride toothpaste, which delivers its effect at the tooth surface, has reduced the significance of the last two mechanisms, which are now thought to play a very minor role.

Key points
- Twice-daily brushing with fluoride toothpaste is an effective preventive measure, but requires compliance. *Evidence Base A*

- A small pea-sized amount of fluoride toothpaste should be used by young children (a small smear for babies) and brushing with fluoride toothpaste should be supervised. *Evidence Base C*

- Water fluoridation is safe and effective, but should be targeted at communities with higher caries levels where it is technically feasible. *Evidence Base A*

- Fluoride supplements, though shown to be effective in clinical trials, may not be as effective in practice for home use or in community schemes. *Evidence Base B*

Diet and oral health

3

Sugars and dental caries

The evidence for a link between sugars and caries comes from a variety of sources. Epidemiological studies have demonstrated a clear correlation between caries experience and mean sugars consumption levels in different countries. When communities have shown changes in sugars consumption, such as during World War II (1939–1945) when consumption fell, a corresponding fall in caries prevalence has been observed. Similarly, groups having low or restricted sugars consumption and those with high consumption of sugars, show corresponding lower or higher levels of caries experience. Children using sugars-sweetened medicines over long periods have shown higher caries levels compared to a control group. Human clinical studies have demonstrated that, when sugars consumption is increased under controlled conditions, then the caries increment follows and it falls when consumption is reduced. Laboratory studies have demonstrated, by the use of miniature pH electrodes inserted into the plaque on teeth, an immediate fall in pH on the application of a neutral sugar solution, with the acidity persisting for 20 minutes to two hours.

Sugars in food and drinks

The sugars most responsible for dental caries have been classified by the Committee on Medical Aspects of Food Policy (now the Scientific Advisory Committee on Nutrition) as *non-milk extrinsic sugars* (NMES),[6] as illustrated in Figure 3.1.

NMES are those which are added to food and drinks during processing, manufacture or preparation. NMES also include sugars naturally present in fresh fruit juices, honey and syrups. The reason that NMES are implicated is that they are simple sugars that can rapidly enter the plaque bacteria and be converted to acid and are often frequently consumed in amounts far in excess of nutritional needs. Sugars naturally present in fruit and vegetables – and

19

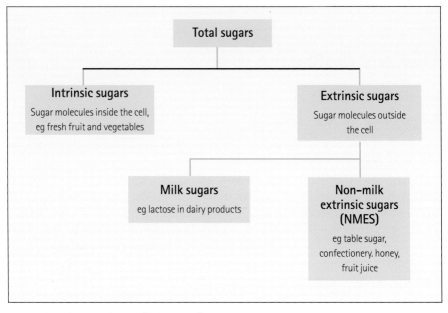

Fig. 3.1 Classification of sugars (COMA, 1989).

eaten as such – are not considered to be cariogenic. This is because they are contained within the cell structure of the plant and may not be fully released into the mouth during eating. Fruit and vegetables are an essential part of a healthy diet. Concentrated fruit juices and dried fruits have a high concentration of sugars. While these are included within the fruit and vegetables recommended by the '5 a day' programme, sponsored by the Department of Health in England, from a dental perspective their frequent consumption especially between meals could increase the risk of caries. It should be noted that fresh fruit juices and dried fruit, irrespective of how much is consumed, may each only constitute one of the five daily portions and this point should be stressed when giving dietary advice. Lactose, the sugar in milk, is less cariogenic than other dietary sugars. When naturally present in milk, it appears to be virtually non-cariogenic.

The common non-milk extrinsic dietary sugars are sucrose (refined from beet and cane), glucose, maltose (extracted from many foods) and fructose (extracted from fruit). Fructose is also a NMES when naturally present in natural unsweetened fruit juice, honey and syrups and when used as an additive to foods and drinks. Significant amounts of glucose and fructose are now made industrially from starch. While sucrose is highly cariogenic, animal studies have shown that both glucose and fructose will readily produce caries and combinations of these sugars appear to be as cariogenic as sucrose alone.

Furthermore, there does not appear to be a safe level for sugars concentration in food and drinks, as this is linked in a complex manner with physical consistency. Indeed, in solution, sucrose concentrations below the taste threshold can generate acid in plaque.

Dietary starch, which is a complex carbohydrate, is converted to maltose and glucose in the mouth by enzymes in saliva, and these sugars are then available for metabolizing into acids by plaque bacteria. However, the rate of conversion is slow and dietary starch by itself is very much less important than dietary sugars as a cause of dental caries. Recent research has shown that when starch is cooked at very high temperatures, such as for the production of some snack foods, then the conversion to glucose in the mouth can occur more rapidly.

From a theoretical aspect, sugar-free chewing gum may have a positive benefit for dental health by increasing salivary flow during chewing, which helps to neutralize plaque acid activity. The majority of clinical studies have found a positive benefit.

Cariogenic sugars

Table I Sugars and other compounds added to food and drinks during processing, manufacture or before consumption as sweeteners and that have the potential to cause dental caries.	
glucose*	maltose
fructose*	glucose syrup
hydrolysed starch	maltodextrins
sucrose*	oligofructose

*non-cariogenic when contained in whole fresh fruits, vegetables and grains.

21

Table 2 Products which are essentially a mixture of sugars.	
brown sugar (mainly sucrose)	treacle
maple syrup	honey
golden syrup	

Non-cariogenic sweeteners
These can be classed as either bulk or intense sweeteners.

Table 3 Bulk sweeteners mainly used to add sweetness, calories and bulk to confectionery products.	
maltitol syrup	lactitol
mannitol	xylitol
isomalt	maltitol
sorbitol	

Xylitol
There is considerable evidence from laboratory and clinical studies that xylitol is not only non-cariogenic, but also suppresses the growth of acidogenic bacteria in plaque. There is additional evidence that beneficial effect on the plaque bacteria may be passed from a mother to her children. The use of xylitol in chewing gum has been the subject of a number of extensive clinical trials, which generally have shown a significant caries-inhibiting effect. Xylitol-sweetened chewing gum may provide a benefit for caries prevention.[7]

If consumed in excess, bulk sweeteners can have a laxative effect. While overt diarrhoea is a rare side-effect, children are at greater risk. There is a statutory requirement for these sweeteners to carry the labelling that excessive consumption may produce laxative effects.

Combinations of sugars and intense sweeteners such as saccharin are used in some products; however the latter will not have a protective role and such products must be classified as cariogenic. Concentrated soft drinks, which are the main source of artificial sweeteners in the diet of young children, should be diluted with

Table 4 Intense sweeteners added in small amounts, often to soft drinks.	
Acesulfame K	Aspartame
Saccharin	Cyclamate
Thaumatin	Sucralose
Neohesperidine DC	

extra water for these young consumers to avoid excessive intake. Even if well diluted, such drinks are acidic and have the potential to cause erosion.

It must be remembered that manufacturing problems related to sugars substitution are not just limited to sweetness, cost and safety. Sugars give bulk to many foods and influence properties such as viscosity, texture and shelf life.

The pattern of sugar intake

After consuming sugar, acid is rapidly generated in the dental plaque and, within 1–2 minutes, plaque pH has fallen to levels that favour enamel demineralization. The return to neutrality takes between 20 minutes and two hours, depending on such factors as salivary flow rate and buffering capacity and plaque thickness and composition. Maximum acid production is achieved by modest sugar concentrations, beyond which increased concentrations do not give a greater fall in pH. However, frequent sugar intakes will not allow time for the pH to recover and will prolong the period of plaque acidity. This pattern may allow demineralization to exceed remineralization resulting in a progressive loss of minerals from enamel as illustrated in Figure 1.4a (page 6)

These observations are supported by animal experiments that have shown a direct correlation between sucrose frequency and caries levels.

It has been shown that, in human volunteers who stopped toothbrushing and used two-hourly sucrose rinses, enamel demineralization occurred within three weeks. However, as the amount of NMES consumed has been shown to be independently related to caries experience and as frequency and amount are strongly linked, advice must be to reduce both. This advice is supported by a report from the Committee on Medical Aspects of Food Policy (*Dietary Sugars and Human Disease* 1989).[6]

The frequency and time of consumption of sugars-sweetened foods and drinks have both been shown to be important factors in determining caries levels. Sugars consumed with main meals appear to be of less significance because they are cleared from the mouth by other foods and the high salivary flow rate generated by eating. Other foods taken as part of the meal, such as cheese may help stimulate salivary flow and raise the calcium level in plaque so that remineralization is promoted. However, the same sugars-sweetened items consumed between meals appear to have a much more detrimental effect as well as increasing the total daily frequency count.

Recent research has confirmed that bedtime is the worst time to consume a sugars-sweetened drink or snack. This is due to the low salivary flow rate during sleep and to the fact that toothbrushing is unlikely to remove all traces of any sugary snack taken before bed. Children who consumed both a sugary drink and snack in the hour before bed were found to have four times the number of decayed teeth compared to children who had neither.[8]

Sugars in medicines can also cause decay. Many paediatric medicines, including those sold without prescription, have sugar-free alternatives. Clinicians should prescribe sugar-free medicines and parents/carers should request them. Pharmacists should be encouraged to stock and recommend sugar-free alternatives to the most commonly used prescription and general sale medicines.

Key points
- The frequency and amount of consumption of sugars in drinks and foods are the most important risk factors. *Evidence Base A*

- Sugars-sweetened snacks and drinks should be avoided between meals and especially at bedtime. *Evidence Base B*

- Naturally occurring sugars when consumed in fresh whole fruit, vegetables and cereal grains are not a risk factor for dental caries and these items are an essential part of a healthy balanced diet. *Evidence Base B*

Periodontal diseases

4

While there are a number of diseases, both acute and chronic, that affect the gums and the surrounding bone and fibres that support the teeth, by far the most common are gingivitis and chronic periodontitis. Gingivitis can begin as early as childhood and presents as inflammation of the gum margin, with redness, swelling and bleeding on brushing (Fig. 4.1). Most forms of gingivitis can be reversed by effective oral hygiene. Without adequate personal oral care, a second stage, termed chronic periodontitis can occur. In this stage, which can begin as early as adolescence, the bone and fibres that support the teeth are progressively destroyed (Fig. 4.2). However, the rate of destruction can vary greatly both between and within individuals. This may lead eventually to loosening and finally loss of the tooth, although the process can be slowed by a combination of personal care and professional treatment.

Cause

Periodontal diseases are caused by dental plaque – a soft, sticky film composed mainly of bacteria, which forms on the teeth and is present in all mouths. Bacterial plaque causes a complex response in the individual that the body intends to be protective. However, if the body's immunological defence system

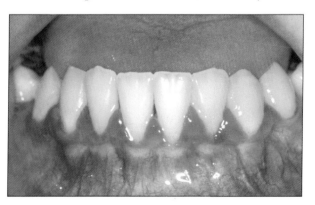

Fig. 4.1 Gingivitis.

25

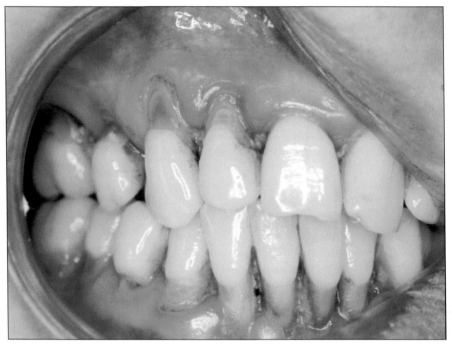

Fig. 4.2 Periodontitis, with abrasion cavities at the necks of teeth caused by incorrect toothbrushing technique.

is not functioning properly, then damage to the periodontal tissues can occur. Similarly, if the amount or virulence of the bacteria increases, then the body's response may not be sufficient to prevent damage. The severity of the damage caused by plaque is determined by a number of factors that fall into two groups – those that cause plaque to be retained on the teeth, and those that modify the nature of the tissue reaction to the bacterial products. The overall balance between the bacterial challenge and the body's response is critical to the maintenance of periodontal health – an upset to the balance (on either side) can result in the development and progression of periodontal disease.

Plaque retention factors
Any irregularity around the teeth will encourage the accumulation of plaque by making tooth cleaning difficult. Such factors include crooked teeth, overhanging edges on fillings, poorly contoured fillings, some types of partial

dentures and calculus. Calculus (tartar) is plaque which has become calcified and hardened and may cause plaque stagnation. Calculus can form above the gum line (supragingival) and below the gum margin (subgingival). As periodontal disease progresses, the shallow space between the gum margin and the tooth deepens to form a periodontal pocket in which plaque and subgingival calculus accumulate.

Modifying factors

There is a strong association between the amount of plaque accumulation and the reaction of the oral tissues. However, variations are seen both in the reaction of the gums and the rate of destruction of the supporting bone. This may be due to a number of factors. The types of bacteria present in plaque vary both between individuals and at different sites within an individual mouth. There is considerable evidence that smoking increases the risk of periodontal disease and reduces the effectiveness of treatment. In many cases, however, the cause of variation is likely to be differences between individuals in the susceptibility of their tooth-supporting structures to the destructive processes caused by bacterial products.

The gum margin around the necks of the teeth is a unique structure in the body as it is an imperfect junction between two quite different body tissues; hard, calcified tooth surface and the soft, vascular tissue of the gums. The body's immunological defence system has to fight a constant battle to prevent harmful bacteria from penetrating this junction and anything that affects this defence system can produce a reaction at the gum margin, usually inflammation. This was first seen as scurvy in seamen before the need for vitamin C was recognized. However, today, a common example is the change produced by the hormonal disturbance during pregnancy, where even modest deposits of plaque can produce a condition known as pregnancy gingivitis. Other systemic conditions that can cause gingival change, often as a first indication, include anaemia, diabetes, HIV/AIDS and leukaemia.

Prevention

As gingivitis precedes adult periodontitis, the main way of limiting periodontal disease is by plaque control directed to maintaining gingival health. This must be considered at two levels – what people can do for themselves by way of plaque control on a daily basis, and what dentists and hygienists/therapists can do to eliminate plaque retention factors and to advise the individual on the most appropriate home care.

What people can do for themselves

The most important plaque control method is effective toothbrushing with a fluoride toothpaste and it should be established as a daily routine from the time of tooth eruption. Toothbrushing skills should be taught to people of all ages. The precise technique is less important than the result, which is that plaque is removed effectively and daily without causing damage to the teeth or gums.

A gentle scrub technique is effective for most people and is easy to teach and readily accepted. Careful use of this method with a recommended type of brush should be encouraged as it will provide effective plaque removal. Most authorities recommend a brush with a small head bearing densely packed soft to medium synthetic filaments. Faulty toothbrushing techniques involving excessive pressure may considerably increase gum recession and loss of tooth substance by mechanical abrasion and must therefore be corrected (see Fig. 4.2).

Plaque-disclosing agents which colour plaque to make it easily visible can be a useful aid to improving plaque control. They will not in themselves remove plaque, but will show areas where plaque remains after brushing. Dental floss and other interdental cleaning aids are of value if used correctly but they will usually require professional advice and instruction. An additional method of plaque control is the use of antiseptics, of which chlorhexidine is the most effective. Although this antiseptic is on general sale in the UK in mouthrinse and gel forms, its tendency to stain teeth and impair taste makes it generally unacceptable for long-term use. Many popular toothpastes contain other chemical plaque-suppressing agents such as triclosan combined with a co-polymer or zinc salts. While these are less effective than chlorhexidine, they do not have the same side-effects and have been shown to be of value to gingival health.

What dental professionals can do

It is the responsibility of the dentist to ensure that any treatment provided minimizes plaque retention; this is a part of treatment planning. Clear advice must be given on the need to clean bridges, dentures and orthodontic appliances (braces) effectively and regularly. Calculus that forms on the teeth above the gum level and within the pockets should be removed regularly by careful professional scaling. While appropriate professional treatment is

28

important, the highest priority should be given to effective daily oral hygiene by the individual.

More information on plaque control can be found in Chapter 5.

Key points
- The risk of developing periodontal disease can be reduced by careful and effective daily toothbrushing. Evidence Base A

- The risk of developing periodontal disease can be reduced by not smoking. Evidence Base B

5 Plaque control and dental diseases

There is ample evidence of an association between plaque and periodontal disease in children and adults. Plaque deposits have been shown to cause gingival inflammation, which is reversed by plaque removal. It follows that plaque control can be endorsed for the prevention of gingivitis, although it should be remembered that once the bone and fibres supporting the tooth have been lost as a result of chronic periodontitis, then plaque control alone is probably insufficient to stabilize the condition. A combination of personal plaque control and professional treatment may then be needed to retard further bone loss.

Based on clinical observation, it had been suggested that dental caries could be controlled by highly effective toothbrushing, without the benefit of fluoride toothpaste. Some research studies have shown that highly efficient toothbrushing techniques can reduce caries. However, plaque removal by normal toothbrushing alone does not appear to be as effective, as some plaque is left in fissures and other stagnation sites where caries occurs, and plaque rapidly begins to reform on cleaned tooth surfaces. For caries prevention, the real value of toothbrushing is now thought to be that it combines plaque removal with the application of fluoride to the tooth surface.

Plaque removal for children

It is generally agreed that most children have insufficient manual dexterity to achieve effective plaque removal with a toothbrush until at least six to seven years of age. Parents should be advised to brush their children's teeth thoroughly twice a day using a small brush. One method of toothbrushing is for the parent to stand behind the child and tilt the child's head upwards so that all tooth surfaces can be brushed using a gentle scrub motion.

Plaque removal for adults

The gentle scrub method of toothbrushing is effective in plaque removal and is easily taught and accepted. It should be carried out with a small toothbrush for ease of access. The method is to place the filaments of the brush at the neck of the tooth and to use very short horizontal movements to dislodge plaque from the stagnation areas at the gum margins around the teeth. The biting surfaces of side and back teeth should then be brushed. Emphasis should be placed on small movements and gentle pressure, together with an unhurried systematic approach to the cleaning of all surfaces. Holding the brush with the fingers in a 'pen' grip may avoid excessive force.

The use of dental floss, mini-brushes and similar interdental cleaning aids can be of great value in individual cases, but specific professional advice and guidance is necessary and care must be taken to avoid damaging the gums. Such aids should be used as an addition to toothbrushing and must not be considered as an alternative.

Recommended toothbrush specifications

While there is a wide variation in toothbrush design, little evidence exists to support specific recommendations. The size of the toothbrush head should be appropriate to the user but it should be remembered that a smaller head will give better access to the back of the mouth and those tooth surfaces that a large-headed brush cannot reach. The filaments (bristles) should be of a synthetic material, round-ended and of a soft-to-medium texture. For children or adults with limited manual dexterity, it can be an advantage to choose a toothbrush with a large handle that provides a firm, comfortable grip. When the bristles become deformed or splayed, plaque removal becomes less effective and the toothbrush should be replaced.

Powered toothbrushes

Modern powered toothbrushes have become very popular. An independent systematic review of existing studies concluded that powered toothbrushes are at least as effective as manual toothbrushes and there is no evidence that they will cause more injuries to the gums than manual brushes.[9] Powered toothbrushes with a rotation oscillation action (ie the head rotates in one direction and then the other) have been shown to be slightly better at removing plaque and reducing gum inflammation than manual toothbrushes, but the long-term benefits are unclear. Some individuals like the 'feel' of powered toothbrushes and they can be helpful in those with limited manual dexterity, such as arthritis sufferers; furthermore, the novelty value in children can encourage compliance with their brushing regime. As with manual toothbrushes, the heads do wear out and need to be replaced regularly.

Chemical plaque suppressants

Of the many agents that have been tested, chlorhexidine has proved to be the most effective plaque suppressant under clinical conditions. It is on general sale in the UK in mouthrinse, gel and spray forms and is used in the management of periodontal disease. It can cause staining of teeth, which is difficult to remove from white fillings and can impair taste. While clinical experience in daily sustained use is limited, two years being the duration of the longest clinical trial reported to date, no other major adverse effects have been reported. Nevertheless, it is generally unacceptable for long-term unsupervised use, one month being the normal limit. It can be of value for short-term use when toothbrushing is difficult or painful, but works best on clean teeth by inhibiting plaque formation.

Other antiseptics without the adverse effects of chlorhexidine are used in many mouthrinses and toothpastes. One of the more effective of these appears to be the phenol derivative, triclosan, when combined with a co-polymer or with zinc compounds. Use of such products may provide benefits to plaque control and gingival health. There is evidence that the non-cariogenic sweetener xylitol inhibits the growth of some plaque bacteria (see page 22). However, its value for the prevention of periodontal disease has not been established.

Key points
- Twice-daily brushing with a manual or powered toothbrush and a fluoride-containing toothpaste is the principal means of plaque control. *Evidence Base A*

- Other aids such as floss and interdental brushes can be highly effective but are best used following professional advice. *Evidence Base C*

6

Erosion

Erosion is the loss of tooth substance caused by the direct action of chemicals on the tooth surface. It is quite different from caries in both appearance and causation. While erosion can occur by chemical action alone, it is sometimes linked to attrition of the teeth due to grinding them, often at night, or eating coarse foods and with abrasion due to excessive brushing with a hard brush or an abrasive toothpaste. Erosion is therefore classed as a type of tooth wear. Indeed, tooth wear in many individuals is due to a combination of attrition, abrasion and erosion in differing proportions.

Clinical presentation

Erosion was described as early as 1892 among Sicilian lemon pickers. The characteristic appearance is loss of enamel and in more severe cases of dentine from specific sites. Erosion should not be confused with caries. While caries affects the surfaces of the teeth where plaque stagnates, erosion affects plaque-free surfaces. Primarily, these are the palatal (inside) aspects of the upper front teeth followed by the labial (lip) aspects of these teeth and the occlusal (biting) surfaces of the premolar (side) and molar (back) teeth (Fig. 6.1). In the deciduous dentition the incisal (biting) edges of the upper front teeth are often lost first (Fig. 6.2).

In the early stages pain is not a feature, but as enamel loss progresses, sensitivity to thermal change and acidic drinks becomes established and more persistent pain can occur in severe cases.

Cause

Erosion is usually due to acids entering the mouth. However cases have been reported amongst workers in the chemical industry and acid battery factories due to atmospheric fumes and from careless use of pipettes in laboratories.

While industrial cases appear to have diminished because of increased awareness in the workplace, two other causes may have become more important. Gastric reflux brings acid into the mouth and is thought to affect

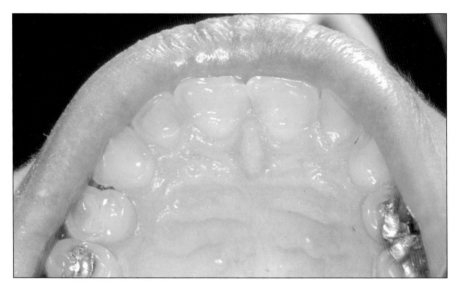

Fig. 6.1 Dental erosion on the palatal aspect of upper anterior teeth. Almost all of the enamel has been lost.

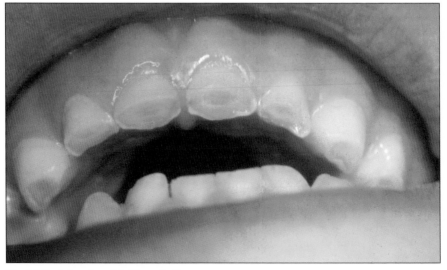

Fig. 6.2 Dental erosion of deciduous teeth.

up to 70% of individuals at some time. Causes include hiatus hernia, pregnancy, motion sickness, alcoholism, obesity and bulimia, of which it can be an early sign. However, dietary factors are thought to be the most common cause today. While citrus fruits have erosive potential, there is little evidence to link the consumption of whole fruit with increased erosion in a normal population.

In contrast, fruit juice is erosive and the frequent consumption of juices has been linked in many reports to increased tooth wear, as have sports-type drinks. Possibly of greater significance is the erosive potential of soft drinks, including carbonated and fruit-based ones. The rapid rise in consumption of fruit juice and soft drinks, following the development of modern containers such as the tetrapak, plastic bottles and aluminium cans, has been blamed for what is generally perceived as an increase in the prevalence of erosion, especially among youngsters. The relationship between frequency of consumption of such drinks and erosion is now established.

The principal ingredient linked to erosion is citric acid, which is found in most fruit juices and soft drinks, however other fruit acids may have an effect. The erosive effect is partly due to its low pH and also because it can demineralize enamel by binding to calcium and removing it from the tooth surface, a process called chelation. Cola-type drinks may also contain phosphoric acid, which produces a low pH. The recent popularity of 'alcopop' type drinks, which are fruit-flavoured alcoholic beverages and strong ciders, all of which have a low pH, has caused concern, but as yet no substantive evidence is available. While the pH of a drink is an indicator of its erosive potential, a measure called total titratable acidity, which gives the capacity of a liquid to dissolve mineral, is a better guide.

However, some other factors are important in determining the risk of erosion. These include the flow rate and buffering capacity of saliva, the manner and frequency of consumption of erosive drinks and the consumption of other foods such as cheese and milk. There is anecdotal evidence that the common habit of swishing carbonated drinks around the mouth before swallowing may increase the danger. In addition, acidic ice lollipops and acid-based sweets may have erosive potential.

At present we lack a universally accepted index for the assessment of erosion and consequently there is no reliable long-term data to indicate changes in the prevalence of erosion over time. However, most clinicians believe that prevalence has increased during the last 20 years. From the many studies in the literature the prevalence of enamel erosion in children appears to vary from less than 10% to 50% according to age. For erosion into dentine the figures are lower, but may affect 25% of children with deciduous teeth. These figures are supported by the 1993 National Child Dental Health Survey.[10] The higher levels usually found in the deciduous dentition are thought to be due to the practice of giving fruit juice in feeding bottles or feeder cups.

Prevention

Erosion can be prevented by reducing the intake of erosive drinks and food. While no safe limit can be established, any reduction is desirable. Children and young adults especially should not have acidic beverages as their main fluid intake. The practices of swishing and frequent sipping of acidic drinks should be discouraged. Taking milk or cheese afterwards may be beneficial. Drinking erosive beverages through a straw has been shown to help, but only if the tip is placed well back in the mouth. It is also sensible to avoid toothbrushing for a period of time after an erosive episode as the brush can damage the softened enamel. There is no conclusive evidence as to how long this should be, but a period of one hour is accepted by most experts.

The resistance of the teeth to erosion can be increased by the use of topical fluorides. Whilst twice daily use of a fluoride toothpaste is considered essential, mouthrinses are also of value. The professional application of fluoride varnishes and gels can give added benefit, both by increasing enamel acid resistance and in reducing sensitivity. In severe cases some form of restoration is usually necessary, often crowns for permanent teeth.

Where gastric regurgitation is suspected because of physical or emotional problems such as bulimia, the patient should be advised to consult their medical practitioner.

Key points
- Limit the frequency of intake of acidic beverages. *Evidence Base B*
- Avoid brushing for one hour after an 'acidic episode'. *Evidence Base C*

Oral cancer

7

Oral tumours

As elsewhere in the body, both benign and malignant tumours can occur in the mouth. Benign tumours tend to be slow growing and localized and are rarely life-threatening. However, malignant tumours can grow rapidly, infiltrate the surrounding area and spread to the lymph glands and other parts of the body, with the formation of secondary or metastatic deposits, especially in the bones, lungs or other organs. If detected early and treated, a complete cure is often possible, but delay makes treatment difficult and approximately half of all cases prove fatal within five years.

Squamous cell carcinoma

The most common type of oral cancer is squamous cell carcinoma which accounts for about 90% of all oral malignancies. They arise from the oral mucosa lining the mouth and covering the tongue. In the majority of cases they present as an ulcer, most commonly in the floor of the mouth, the lateral border of the tongue, or inside the lips. Often they arise within a pre-existing white, red or thickened area of mucosa and at the earliest stage may not show obvious signs of ulceration. Thickened white areas of mucosa, termed leukoplakia, are well recognized as potential sites for malignant change and the appearance of red spots or ulceration within a leukoplakia is often an indication of this change (Fig. 7.1). Malignant ulcers differ from other innocent ulcers by persisting for more than two weeks after any cause is removed. Unlike other forms of oral ulceration, they do not heal or resolve spontaneously. Indeed, any ulcer present for more than three weeks should be investigated without delay.

Other oral tumours

Other tumours can arise in or around the mouth, such as within the jaw bones or from salivary glands, connective tissue, blood vessels or nerves. These

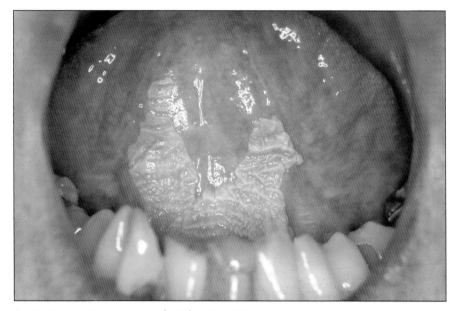

Fig. 7.1 Leukoplakia on the ventral (under) surface of the tongue.

tumours generally present as swellings, but in some cases the first signs may be loosening of teeth, spontaneous fracture of the jaw or enlargement of the lymph glands in the neck.

Prevalence and prognosis

It is estimated that there are about 4,500 new cases of oral cancer each year in the UK, with over 2,000 deaths. The number of cases is increasing and approaches that for cervical cancer, but the overall five-year survival rate is worse and the mortality rate is higher than for most other cancers. For oral cancers detected at the earliest stage, the five-year survival rate is about 90%, but this falls to about 20% for those presenting at the latest stage. The poor overall five-year survival rate is thought to due to the late presentation of many cases. This finding is even more distressing because the mouth is the easiest body cavity to examine. While most cases occur in men, and many cases occur in the over 60s, in recent years there has been a shift towards an earlier age of onset (45–59 years) and an increase in the number of women affected.[11]

Cause and prevention

The main risk factors for oral cancer are tobacco or alcohol and a combination of these factors appears to multiply the risk. The relative risk for long-term smokers who also consume alcohol may be over 30 times greater than non-smokers who are infrequent drinkers. The habits of chewing tobacco and reverse smoking (with the lit end inside the mouth) have been found to be factors, while the common practice amongst some Asian communities of chewing 'betel nut quid', 'paan' or 'ghutka', an addictive blend of tobacco and other vegetable matter, is linked to the high prevalence of oral cancer in the Indian sub-continent and Asian communities in other parts of the world. There is evidence that if smoking ceases then the risk of developing oral cancer falls and about 50% of leukoplakias appear to resolve. Other risk factors include pre-existing white patches on the oral mucosa, including those related to candida infection (see Chapter 8), some viral infections and immuno-suppressive conditions such as AIDS/HIV.

There is evidence that the prevention of many types of malignancy benefit from a higher intake of fresh fruit and vegetables, resulting from their content of vitamin and anti-oxidant compounds. In all cases early diagnosis is vital and argues the case for regular whole mouth examinations and immediate referral of suspicious lesions to an appropriate secondary care clinician.

Key points
- Smoking, other forms of tobacco use and frequent alcohol consumption are the main risk factors. *Evidence Base A*

- White or red patches and oral ulceration present for more than three weeks require immediate investigation. *Evidence Base C*

- Smokers who wish to give up should be given appropriate support to do so. *Evidence Base C*

8

Other oral diseases

There are a number of other conditions that can develop in the mouth and require professional advice and help.

Oral candidosis

Infection with the fungus *Candida albicans* can present in the mouth in many forms, both acute and chronic. The most common presentations are *angular chelitis*, a chronic infection of the angles of the mouth, usually seen in older people, especially those with old, worn dentures (Fig. 8.1) and *denture sore mouth* a chronic infection usually seen in the palate where a denture is worn at night, instead of being removed as generally advised (Fig. 8.2). Some cases are associated with poor nutrition, chronic anaemia, diabetes or depression of the immune system as in AIDS/HIV infection. Prevention of these common forms depends on treating any systemic factors and the removal and thorough cleaning of dentures each night and replacement when they are worn out (see Chapter 10).

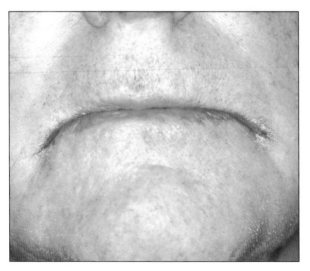

Fig. 8.1 Angular chelitis, a form of chronic Candida infection.

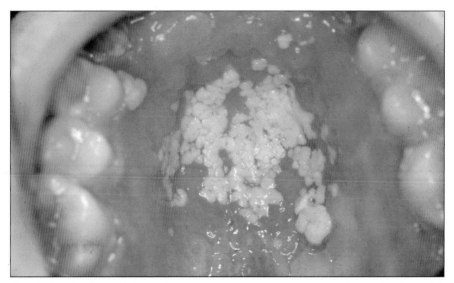

Fig. 8.2 Candida infection in the palate associated with poor hygiene practice in the wearing of a partial upper denture. The yellow clumps are colonies of Candida organisms growing on the mucosa.

Oral ulceration

About 25% of the population suffers from *minor apthous ulceration* – the common mouth ulcer – on a regular basis. The ulcers occur either singly or in small crops, often inside the lips or cheek and heal with or without treatment within 10 days. The cause remains unknown, although some cases are associated with systemic illness such as anaemia or diabetes. A more severe form, *major apthous ulceration*, generally produces solitary ulcers, which take up to a month to heal, often leaving a residual scar.

Herpes simplex infection can cause a common form of oral ulceration. Viral in origin, it can produce a very sore mouth with crops of small grey ulcers, that generally heal spontaneously within 10 days. The primary infection can occur in infancy and may be confused with teething. When young children are affected, they can become rapidly dehydrated and an adequate fluid intake is essential. As the virus often remains dormant in the tissues, secondary attacks can occur, either in the mouth or on the lips as *herpes labalis* or *cold sores*.

Ulceration can also be caused by trauma, such as lip biting or by the sharp edge of a denture, however all innocent ulcers should heal within a month.

White and red patches

A number of conditions can present as white or red patches in the mouth. Some patches can be caused by simple friction from cheek biting, but others may be forms of chronic candidosis or premalignant conditions. Any white or red patch persisting for more than a few weeks should be investigated.

Dry mouth

Xerostomia, or dry mouth, is a common condition that can make eating or even speech difficult and can increase the risk of dental caries and periodontal disease. Although it can affect people of all ages, it appears to be more common in the elderly. However, recent research suggests that age, in itself, is not an important factor, but possibly the wide range of drugs that induce xerostomia as a side-effect and which many elderly people require. Specific causes of xerostomia include diabetes, a blocked salivary duct, chronic dehydration and more rarely, a salivary gland tumour or Sjögrens syndrome. A very severe form of xerostomia can follow from radiotherapy for tumours of the head or neck, as salivary glands are very sensitive to radiation. Rapidly progressive dental caries and periodontal disease can quickly follow and this condition requires the intensive application of preventive measures. Apart from treating any basic cause, artificial saliva can be used, but many sufferers find that the frequent sipping of iced water gives the best relief. Spicy foods should be avoided, however chewing sugar-free gum may provide relief.

There are some conditions arising elsewhere in the body that can have a visible effect within the mouth, such as pregnancy, anaemia and HIV infection (AIDS). These also need professional advice and help.

Key points
- Oral candidosis, when not associated with dentures, may be a sign of systemic disease causing immunosupression. *Evidence Base B*

- Dentures should be removed and cleaned every night and should be replaced when damaged, ill-fitting or worn out. *Evidence Base C*

Advice for children under five

9

Toothbrushing

Regular, twice daily, toothbrushing with a fluoride toothpaste can be introduced shortly after the appearance of the first teeth. However, in the Republic of Ireland, because of widespread water fluoridation, the advice is to begin brushing from two years of age, or use a non-fluoride toothpaste before two years. A small, soft toothbrush should be used, with just a smear of toothpaste, increasing from the age of about three years, to a small pea-sized amount for children under seven years. A gentle and systematic approach should be used with the aim of cleaning the outside, inside and biting surfaces of all teeth, including the back ones when they appear, usually between one and two years of age. Younger children are often quite happy to brush their own teeth, but lack the manual dexterity to do so efficiently. Parents should supervise or assist with brushing until the children can do it effectively, usually by the age of seven years. However, some children need supervision beyond this age.

A fluoride toothpaste is recommended. Low fluoride toothpastes provide only limited anticaries benefit and unless the child and any siblings are caries-free and in good health, a regular family fluoride toothpaste should be used. However, care should be taken to ensure that younger children do not eat toothpaste directly from the tube or swallow excessive amounts from the brush.

Drinks

Parents and carers of infants should be specifically warned against the practice of allowing prolonged drinking from a bottle, valve-type feeder or any other type of lidded feeder cup of any sugars-sweetened drink, including carbonated drinks, fruit-based juices, squash and natural fruit juice. The prolonged contact time between the sugar in the drink and the teeth is well recognized as a cause of rapidly progressing decay, usually of the upper front teeth, resulting in a condition, previously referred to as 'nursing bottle caries', but now termed 'early childhood caries' (Fig. 9.1). The risk from this practice is increased if the bottle

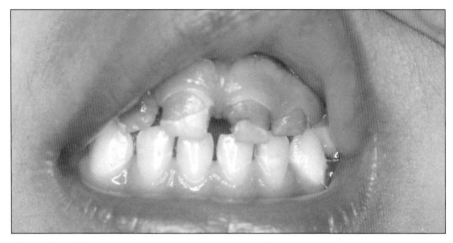

Fig. 9.1 Early childhood caries, better known as 'bottle caries'.

is used to comfort the child, especially at bedtime or when in a cot or pushchair.

If sugars-sweetened drinks are given to younger children, they should be very well diluted, taken preferably at meal times only and drinking times should be kept short. An open cup or beaker should be used, never a bottle. Preferable alternatives are the lightly flavoured mineral waters, which state that they are suitable for infants. Parents and carers should be aware however that the sugar content of some flavoured bottled mineral waters can be as high as 10% and the precautions given above for sugars-sweetened drinks should be followed. A child's normal fluid intake should ideally be plain water or milk.

Breast milk is the best form of nutrition for infants. When breastfeeding is not possible, cows' milk formulas are the preferred option. Infants and children should continue on hydrolyzed protein infant formulas or soya infant formulas until they are two years old. Hydrolyzed protein infant formulas are better nutritionally than those based on soya and infants with an allergy to cows' milk may also have an allergy to soya formula. However, mothers who have been advised by their GP or other health professional to feed their baby soya-based infant formulas, should continue to do so. Soya-based infant formulas contain sugars that can cause tooth decay, so it will be particularly important to be careful about caring for the baby's teeth once they start coming through.

Key points

- Parents should supervise or assist with brushing until children can do it effectively, usually by the age of seven years. *Evidence Base C*

- Low-fluoride toothpastes provide only limited anticaries benefit. *Evidence Base A*

- A child's normal fluid intake should ideally be plain water or milk. *Evidence Base C*

10

Advice for denture wearers and older people

While the number of denture wearers, especially full dentures, has steadily declined, it is estimated that by 2018, around 5% of the adult population will be edentulous and need full dentures (approximately two million people in the UK); a combination of natural teeth and dentures will still be as common as ever for the next 20 years. Demographic changes suggest an increasing proportion of these will be elderly and living either alone, possibly receiving community care, or in residential care or nursing care homes. The dental state of people in residential care is often poor, because help needed with oral hygiene may not be available. It is important that the wearers of full or partial dentures, and especially their carers, understand the need for special care if the health of their mouths and any remaining teeth are to be safeguarded.

Denture cleaning

Routine care should include cleaning of the dentures after every meal and before going to bed. Ideally all dentures should be removed before sleeping to allow the soft tissues of the mouth to recover from the denture-bearing load and to remove the risk of injury or *Candida* infection. Where this is not practical, they should be removed for at least four hours during the day. A small, soft brush and a denture cleaning paste or liquid soap should be used to clean all denture surfaces before rinsing the denture and placing it in a hypochlorite-based soaking solution of the *Steradent* type. Hypochlorite is bactericidal and fungicidal and helps to break down the organic matrix of adherent plaque that forms on the dentures, but can cause bleaching of denture plastic if dentures are soaked for long periods or in hot water. Hypochlorite is not suitable for metal-based dentures for which special soaking solutions containing alkaline peroxide are available. After soaking, the dentures should be brushed and rinsed with water before being inserted. With all cleaning and soaking agents, manufacturer's instructions should be carefully followed. It should be stressed that soaking alone will not clean dentures and thorough brushing before soaking is essential. Any natural teeth should be brushed twice daily with a fluoride toothpaste. The roof of the mouth, the gum ridges and tongue should be gently cleaned daily with a soft brush to remove any food particles and plaque.

Dentures, whether full or partial, do not last indefinitely. The ridges progressively change shape and the edges of the dentures can then begin to irritate the surrounding mucosa. This may cause the dentures to become loose or painful to wear. Even if they remain comfortable, the plastic teeth on the dentures wear down, causing the vertical height between nose and chin to be reduced and the lips to fall in. Often, dentures can be improved by relining the fitting surface, but sometimes older people do not take well to completely new dentures. However, if badly worn, broken or ill-fitting they should be replaced.

Because of these considerations, it is advised that denture wearers have their mouths and dentures examined at least every year. As the loss of a denture may cause great distress, especially for older people, dentists making dentures should be asked to include an embedded identification name.

Root caries

An increasing number of elderly people are retaining some or all of their natural teeth. Since many will have periodontal disease with gum recession, caries may develop on the exposed root surfaces. This is a common problem, made worse by reduced salivary flow and difficulty in maintaining good plaque control, especially round lower anterior teeth. Treating root caries can be difficult, especially in lower anterior teeth, but poor oral hygiene, possibly aggravated by ill-fitting partial dentures and periodontal disease, in an institutionalized elderly person in poor health, can result in a major clinical problem. For home care, careful and effective toothbrushing with a high concentration fluoride toothpaste is recommended, together with regular dental check-ups. If teeth are sensitive to hot and cold drinks, the use of a fluoride-containing 'sensitive toothpaste' can give relief. However, if discomfort persists, then dental advice should be sought. The use of interdental brushes, especially for cleaning between the lower anterior teeth can be beneficial, but again dental advice should be sought.

Apart from problems related to teeth, gums and dentures, the elderly are more prone to dry mouth, possibly linked to their medication and *Candida* infections of the mouth. It must be remembered that the majority of oral cancers occur in the over 60s. The proper dental care of the elderly, especially those in residential care homes, is increasingly a cause for concern. Oral health education for community care, residential and nursing care workers should be a part of their training and should be coordinated with local dental services.

Key points
- Everyone, including those with full dentures should have regular oral examinations. *Evidence Base C*

- Dentures should be removed and cleaned every night and should be replaced when damaged, ill-fitting or worn out. *Evidence Base C*

Frequency of oral examinations

11

While it is accepted that oral examinations at appropriate intervals are of value in maintaining oral health, there is little evidence to support a specific interval or to quantify the benefit and no evidence that six-monthly recalls are the optimum frequency.[12] There are now very many children and adults with little or no dental disease for whom frequent attendance is inappropriate. However, in some areas and among some social groups, the level of oral disease remains high while frequency of attendance is low.

The maintenance of periodontal health depends upon daily personal plaque control. Regular professional care may be required at intervals depending on the needs of the individual. With respect to decay, once a definite cavity is present, it cannot be remineralized, but the tooth can be restored and the importance of early detection and appropriate treatment makes dental attendance advisable. Other disorders can occur in the mouth which are unrelated to the presence of natural teeth and which may be life-threatening.

For all of these reasons, the period between oral examinations must be flexible and based on a professional assessment of the risk from oral disease. The period between oral examinations for everyone, irrespective of age or dental condition, should be about one year. This period can be extended for adults with no evidence of dental disease, who are in good general health and do not use tobacco and have low and infrequent sugar and alcohol consumption. Children may need to be seen more frequently, as may those who are at increased risk to oral disease because of smoking, medical, physical or social factors, or for whom dental treatment presents difficulties because of their medical or physical condition. Attendance will enable the health of the whole mouth to be monitored and appropriate dental health advice and early treatment to be provided when needed.

Key points

- There is no evidence that six-monthly recalls are the optimum frequency. E*vidence Base C*

- Most people, irrespective of age and dental condition should have an oral examination about once a year. *Evidence Base C*

- The period between examinations should be determined on dental advice and reflect the individual risk of oral disease and medical, physical and social factors. *Evidence Base C*

12

Health education

What is health education?

There are many definitions of health education, however one of the most useful is an adaptation of a definition from the World Health Organization, '*Health education is the process by which people are given information to enable them to exercise a greater degree of control over their own health*'.

The process of formulating and delivering health education messages includes a series of steps.

- The first step is to gain an understanding of the basic cause of the disease process under consideration. Taking dental caries as an example, the basic mechanism is the conversion of sugars in the diet into acid by the bacteria in plaque on the surfaces of the teeth.

- Next it is necessary to identify the essential causative factors. Some of these will be beyond individual personal control, such as genetically linked or environmental factors. However, others may be under the control of the individual and amenable to change. In the case of caries, factors under personal control can include the effective use of fluoride toothpaste and the frequency of consumption of sugar-containing foods and drinks.

- The third stage is to agree scientifically based and socially acceptable messages for the public aimed at encouraging beneficial behavioural changes. For the prevention of dental caries one scientifically sound message would be that people should never consume sugars as part of their diet. However, compliance with this message is quite unrealistic because sugars are present in many foods and drinks, either naturally or artificially added. A more sensible message is to avoid sugars-sweetened food and drink between meals and at bedtime. This message can reduce the risk from tooth decay and is more likely to be accepted, though it may need to be modified further where individuals' eating patterns do not conform to traditional mealtimes, and there may be no regular fixed bedtime for children.

- The final, and possibly the most difficult stage of oral health education is that of communication. This process aims to ensure that key information is conveyed comprehensibly to the right target audience, in the right context, at the right time. In line with the World Health Organization's Ottawa Charter, strategic aims for health promotion include traditional methods of health education, such as giving information and advice, thereby developing personal knowledge and skills. However, health promotion may also include other elements: building public policies that support health; creating supportive environments; strengthening community action; and re-orientating health services. These are beyond the scope of this book, but vital if health education initiatives are to be successful.

Does health education work?

One of the most debated issues in public health is the effectiveness of health education and promotion. Much public money is spent on a range of interventions, ranging from one-to-one advice in the GP surgery, to comprehensive healthy schools schemes, and mass media campaigns aimed for example at encouraging smoking cessation. The strength of the evidence-base for these interventions varies. A number of systematic reviews have examined studies in the dental field. Their findings were not always consistent, however the following conclusions were published in the report commissioned by Health Promotion Wales.[13]

- There is clear evidence that oral health education/promotion can be effective in bringing about changes in people's knowledge, and in improving people's oral health.
- It is unclear whether one-off oral health promotion initiatives are sufficient to improve individuals' oral health significantly for long periods.
- There is evidence that programmes using more innovative approaches than the medical/behavioural model, have more potential for longer-term

behaviour changes. They are more likely to be based on models of education and health behaviour which recognize the full variety of factors which influence a person's ability to comply with any messages given.

- Limited short-term behaviour changes are achievable using simple persuasive approaches. Greater or longer-term changes appear possible by using more tailored approaches that are based around active participation and addressing social, cultural and personal norms and values. The use of appropriate language and simple messages is important in avoiding confusion.

- Some studies show that health education which targets whole populations may increase inequalities in health.

- Preventive and comprehensive clinical approaches (including the appropriate use of fissure sealants) to oral health education can be effective in reducing the incidence of dental caries. However, this approach is intensive, and may not reach those in greatest need.

- Changing personal health behaviour appears to be more difficult for some groups than others; this may result in blaming the victim for not making the appropriate behaviour changes.

- Fluoride toothpaste is an important and effective method of delivering fluoride, although it will not reach the entire population. Evidence for the effectiveness of fluoride supplements, such as fluoride tablets, in home use and community schemes is at best equivocal and often shows them to be ineffective.

The Health Education Authority's review[14] concluded that:

- Oral health promotion, which includes the use of therapeutic agents incorporating fluoride (whether in the form of toothpaste, tablets, drops, gels or rinses) is effective in reducing the development of caries. These improvements are cumulative and increase over time. Daily brushing with fluoride toothpaste is easier to achieve than regular use of other fluoride supplements. There is no evidence that oral health promotion *per se* affects caries rates, even if changes in behaviour are achieved, unless fluoride is being used.

- Clinical chairside advice and instruction aimed at improving oral hygiene have been demonstrated to be effective.

- Oral health education on an individual level aimed at improving oral hygiene is capable of reducing plaque levels. However, there is strong evidence that changes achieved are short-term and are not sustained. Interventions are effective even when very simple direct instruction is used. Cognitive-behavioural techniques are not required in order to achieve changes in plaque levels.

- The evidence suggests that oral health promotion is effective in increasing knowledge levels, but there is no evidence that changes in knowledge are causally related to changes in behaviour. However, there would appear to be an ethical responsibility for scientific knowledge to be disseminated to the public, irrespective of what the population does with that knowledge.

- Attempts to control individuals' consumption of sweet foods and drinks are generally not satisfactorily evaluated. However, when such interventions are directed at individuals, they appear to be of limited value.

In an age when cost-benefit assumes growing importance in healthcare, the effectiveness of oral health education in terms of the reduction in disease and healthcare costs is clearly of great significance, when investing scarce resources. However, there is also an ethical obligation for health professionals possessing information that could reduce the prevalence of disease to inform the public accordingly, irrespective of whether a cost benefit can be proven to follow. The right of individuals to health education information was clearly defined by the Ottawa Charter in 1987.

Therefore, three things are clear. Firstly, that more research is needed with the aims of improving the quality of health education delivered and evaluating the results of interventions, including their sustainability. The second is that although strong evidence for the effectiveness of health education and promotion is lacking in some areas, this does not remove from health professionals the responsibility to provide the public with all available information for the promotion of good health. Finally, in order to be effective, health education needs to be properly planned and organized, using the skills of the whole dental team, and the best quality and most appropriate resources.

Which topics are included in this document?

Over the years, many requests had been received to include additional topics within *The Scientific Basis of Dental Health Education* document. To understand the problems involved in selecting topics for inclusion, it is helpful to consider possible topics under three headings.

- Topics where a substantial body of scientific evidence is available to support a useful health education statement. An example being the use of fluoride toothpaste.

- Topics where guidance for the public in the form of a health education message is required but where scientific evidence is lacking. Provided that there is a consensus of scientific opinion, a statement can be made, though this will be subject to change as new evidence and guidelines are published. An example being how often people should have a dental check-up.

- Topics that require guidance for the public but where there is neither a substantial body of scientific evidence nor a consensus of opinion amongst experts. If experts cannot agree then no statement can or should be given. An example is whether the teeth should be brushed before or after eating.

The nature of scientific evidence

Scientific evidence comes in many forms, but in the context of oral health it breaks down and into two main categories:

Laboratory-based studies
These range from purely chemical or biological observations and experiments on the structure of teeth and the mouth, to experiments involving animals or small groups of human volunteers. Examples include the analysis of the changes that occur in teeth when they decay, and studies on the effect on bacteria in the mouth when human volunteers use different types of toothpaste.

Clinical studies

These include observational studies where existing aspects of health are studied in large groups or populations without any form of intervention. These studies can include longitudinal ones where a group of subjects are followed over a period of time, cross-sectional studies and case-controlled studies where a comparison is made with a control group. An important type of clinical study is the interventional experiment. These studies are usually made up of at least two groups, one of which will be a control group who received no intervention and the other groups will follow some form of experimental regime. A good example is the clinical trial of a new toothpaste. In an ideal experiment, subjects will be randomly allocated to a group and the research workers who make the observations will have no knowledge of the group to which any subject has been allocated. This type of experiment is called a *randomized controlled trial* (RCT) and has often been described as the gold standard for clinical research.

Good research studies are usually published in peer-reviewed scientific and clinical journals. These accept only those manuscripts which have been independently reviewed and refereed by experts in the field to ensure that the methods used and the conclusion that have been drawn are valid. A very useful overview of research in any particular field is often provided by a *systematic review*. This is usually written by leading experts who look at all the research that has been done, compare and contrast the results, possibly commenting on the quality of the research and draw appropriate conclusions. Finally, there is a method of comparing the results from a number of studies that have looked at the same issue, usually in the form of randomized controlled trials. Using a sophisticated statistical analysis, the results from all of the trials are pooled together to arrive at one conclusion. This type of overall analysis of results is called a *meta-analysis*.

One very important point must be made about the result of any scientific research. When the conclusion of a study is that '*there is no evidence to form a conclusion*', it does not mean that the negative situation has been firmly established. It simply means that the experiment has not provided evidence for or against the relationship being studied. This is a point that is frequently misunderstood by those without a scientific background, who will reasonably assume that when a scientist says that there is no evidence for this or that, it means that it is not true. All the scientist is saying is that the experiment does not give any evidence to draw a conclusion. It is possible that next week or next year evidence will appear that does establish the case.

Health education and evidence-based dentistry

From the early 1970s there has been a growing interest in placing all aspects of clinical practice on an evidence-supported basis. One of the pioneers of this movement was Professor Archie Cochrane, who gave his name to an international collaborative network of groups with the aim of developing evidence-based decision-making for clinical interventions. The Cochrane Network produces a series of systematic reviews of scientific evidence on a range of topics and some of these are used to support statements made in this document. A further extension of this movement is the appearance of a number of organizations and networks whose aim is to standardize and integrate the methods used for the development of guidelines for clinical practice. In the United Kingdom one of the most useful is that developed by the Scottish Inter-collegiate Guidelines Network (www.sign.ac.uk). One result of this work has been to establish a framework that enables those involved in producing clinical guidelines to formulate them on a common basis.

The concept of putting clinical practice on to an evidence basis has run in parallel with work to ensure that health education messages given to the public are based on sound scientific evidence. Nevertheless, an important difference between these two areas is that while the evidence for clinical interventions ideally comes from high quality clinical studies such as a randomized controlled trials (RCT), the evidence to support dental health education messages often comes from laboratory-based studies. Because of this difference, a grading system for evidence relating to clinical interventions is not appropriate for grading the quality of evidence in relation to health education issues. A complex system for indicating levels of evidence has been developed by the Centre for Evidence-based Medicine in Oxford (CEM) and this scheme is undergoing constant refinement (www.ihs.ox.ac.uk/cebd). In this book, a simple scheme is introduced to give an indication of the volume and quality of evidence supporting key statements for dental health education and is referred to as *Evidence Bases*. The equivalent nearest CEM levels are given in brackets.

- *Level A:* Statements supported by meta-analyses or systematic reviews. (CEM levels 1 and 2)

- *Level B:* Statements supported by the majority of relevant research studies. (CEM level 3 and 4)

- *Level C:* Statements that cannot be supported by a substantial body of research evidence, but where there is a consensus of scientific and professional opinion to support the statement. There may nevertheless be dissenting views, as the issue may be the subject of continuing debate and ongoing research studies. (CEM level 5)

Where appropriate these grades are marked as *Evidence Bases A, B* and *C,* respectively.

Key points

- Health education includes giving people personally relevant information about their health, which is based on a consensus of scientific evidence and opinion. *Evidence Base C*

- We have a responsibility to base health education programmes on the best available evidence of what works, and to evaluate interventions in order to strengthen the evidence-base and improve the quality of health education. *Evidence Base C*

Further Reading

(in alphabetical order)

Blinkhorn A. Oral health education. *In* Seward M H, Rothwell P S (eds) *Oral health promotion with Teamwork*. Sheffield: Teamwork Publications, 1997.

Clarkson J, Harrison J E, Ismail A I, Needleman I, Worthington H. *Evidence Based Dentistry for Effective Practice*. London: Martin Dunitz, 2003.

The Dairy Council. *Topical Update: Diet and Dental Health*. London: The Dairy Council, 2001.

Davies R M, Davies G M, Ellwood R P. Prevention. Part 4: Toothbrushing: what advice should be given to patients? *Br Dent J* 2003; **195**: 135–141.

Daly B, Watt R G, Batchelor P, Treasure E T. *Essential Dental Public Health*. Oxford: OUP, 2002.

Department of Health. *Dietary sugars and human disease*. Report of the Committee on Medical Aspects of Food Policy [COMA]. London: HMSO, 1989.

Department of Health. *Weaning and The Weaning Diet*. Report of the Working Group on the Weaning Diet of the Committee on Medical Aspects of Food Policy [COMA]. London: HMSO, 1994

Department of Health (1997). Statement on Sugar, formulated by COMA. Published in *Food Safety Information Bulletin*, and available at www.doh.gov.uk/coma/state.htm.

Department of Health. Modernising NHS Dentistry. In *Implementing the NHS Plan*. London: HMSO, 2000.

Fejerskov O, Nyvad B, Kidd E A M. Clinical and histological manifestations of dental caries. *In* Fejerskov O, Kidd E A M (eds) *Dental caries the disease and its clinical management*. pp 71–98 Oxford: Blackwell Munksgaard, 2003.

Health Development Agency. *Standard for training in smoking cessation treatments*. London: Health Development Agency, 2003.

Health Education Authority. *Sugars in the diet*. London: Health Education Authority, 1999.

Health Technology and Assessment NHS R & D HTA Programme report on The clinical effectiveness and cost-effectiveness of routine dental checks: a systematic review and economic evaluation, by Davenport C, Elley K, Salas C, Taylor-Weetman C L, Fry-Smith A, Bryan S, Taylor R. Executive Summary, *Health Technology Assessment* 2003; Vol 7: No 7.

Holbrook W P, Arnadottir I B. Prevention. Part 3: Prevention of tooth wear. *Br Dent J* 2003; **195**: 75–81.

Jenkins, W M M, Heasman P A The prevention and control of periodontal disease. *In* Murray J J, Nunn J H, Steele J G (eds) *The Prevention of Oral Disease*. 4th edn, pp 123–144. Oxford: Oxford Medical Publications, 2003.

Kent G, Croucher R. *Achieving Oral Health: the social context of dental care*. Oxford: Wright, 1998.

Marinho V C, Higgins J P, Sheiham A, Logan S. Fluoride toothpastes for preventing dental caries in children and adolescents (Cochrane Review). Cochrane Database Syst Rev. 2003;(1):CD002278.

Moynihan P J. Dietary advice in dental practice. *Br Dent J* 2002; **193**: 563–568.

Moynihan P J. Diet and dental caries. *In* Murray J J, Nunn J H, Steele J G (eds) *The Prevention of Oral Disease*. 4th edn, pp. 10-34. Oxford: Oxford Medical Publications, 2003.

Murray J J, Rugg-Gunn, A J, Jenkins, G N. *Fluorides in caries prevention*. 3rd edn., Oxford: Butterworth-Heinemann, 1991.

Nuttal N, Steele J G, Nunn J, *et al*. *A Guide to the UK Adult Dental Health Survey 1998*. London: BDJ Books, 2001.

Palmer R T M, Floyd P D. Periodontology: a clinical approach, 3: Non-surgical treatment and maintenance, *Br Dent J* 1995; **178**: 263–268.

Pine C. (ed). *Community Oral Health*. Oxford: Wright, 1997.

Royal College of Physicians of London. *Fluoride, teeth and health*. Tunbridge Wells: Pitman Medical, 1976.

Rugg-Gunn A J, Nunn J. *Nutrition, Diet and Oral Health*. Oxford: Oxford University Press, 1999.

Sheiham A. Dietary effects on dental diseases. *Public Health Nutrition* 2001: **4**(2b); 569–591.

Sutcliffe P. Oral cleanliness and dental caries. *In* Murray J J (ed) *The Prevention of Dental Disease*. 3rd edn, pp. 68–77. Oxford: Oxford Medical Publications, 1996.

Steele J, Walls A. Prevention in the ageing population. *In* Murray J J, Nunn J H, Steele J G (eds) *The Prevention of Oral Disease*. 4th edn, pp 190–207. Oxford: Oxford Medical Publications, 2003.

ten Cate J M, Imfeld T (eds) Etiology, mechanism and implications of dental erosion. *European J Oral Sci* 1996; **104**:(2, Pt. 2).

Watt R G, Daly B. Prevention. Part 1: Smoking cessation advice within the general dental practice. *Br Dent J* 2003; **194**: 665–668.

Watt R G, McGlone P. Prevention. Part 2: Dietary advice in the dental surgery. *Br Dent J* 2003; **195**: 27–31.

West R, McNeill A, Raw M. Smoking cessation guidelines for health professionals: an update. *Thorax* 2000; **55**: 987–999.

WHO. Diet in the Prevention of Chronic disease. Technical Report Series 916. Geneva: WHO, 2003.

References

1. Pitts N B, Boyles J J, Nugent Z J. The dental caries experience of 5-year-old children in England and Wales. Surveys co-ordinated by the British Association for the Study of Community Dentistry in 2001/2002. *Community Dent Health* 2003; **20**: 49–54.

2. Pitts N B, Evans D J, Nugent Z J. The dental caries experience of 5-year-old children in the United Kingdom. Surveys co-ordinated by the British Association for the Study of Community Dentistry in 1997/98. *Community Dent Health* 1999; **16**: 50–56.

3. Pine C, Burnside G, Craven R. Inequalities in dental health in the North-West of England. *Community Dent Health* 2003; **20**: 53–54.

4. Holt R D, Nunn J H, Rock W P, Page J. Fluoride Dietary Supplements and fluoride toothpaste for children. *Int J Paed Dent* 1996; **6**: 139–142.

5. NHS Centre for Reviews and Dissemination. *Fluoridation of Drinking Water: a Systematic Review of its Efficacy and Safety* (Report No 18). York: University of York, 2000.

6. Department of Health. *Dietary sugars and human disease* — Report of the Committee on Medical Aspects of Food Policy [COMA]. London: HMSO, 1989.

7. Maguire A, Rugg-Gunn A J. Xylitol and caries prevention – is it a magic bullet? *Br Dent J* 2003; **194**: 429–438.

8. Levine R S. Caries experience and bedtime consumption of sugar-sweetened foods and drinks – a survey of 600 children. *Community Dent Health* 2001; **18**: 228–231.

9. Heanue M, Deacon S A, Deery C, Robinson P G, Walmsley A D, Worthington H V, Shaw W C. Manual versus powered toothbrushing for oral health (Cochrane Review) Cochran Library, 2003. Issue 1. Oxford: Update Software.

10. O'Brian M. *Child Dental Health in the United Kingdom 1993*. Office of Population Census and Surveys. London: HMSO, 1994.

11. Cancer Research UK (2003) www.cancerresearchuk.org

12. Davenport C F, Elley K M, Fry-Smith A, Taylor-Wheetman C L, Taylor R S. The effectiveness of routine dental checks; a systematic review of the evidence base. *Br Dent J* 2003; **195**: 87–98.

13. Sprod A J, Anderson A, Treasure E T. *Effective oral health promotion: Literature review*. Technical Report 20. Cardiff: Health Promotion Wales, 1996.

14. Kay E J, Locker D. *Effectiveness of oral health promotion: a review*. London: Health Education Authority, 1997.

Appendix 1

Smoking cessation and the dental team

Smoking remains the greatest preventable cause of disease and early death in England, and one of the greatest causes of the health divide between rich and poor. It is an addictive behaviour with strong social associations and is very difficult to stop. Overall, the government aims to persuade smokers to give up, to aid them in doing so, and to persuade non-smokers, particularly children, not to start. Smoking cessation interventions delivered through the NHS are an extremely cost effective way of preserving life and reducing ill health. GPs and practice nurses should receive training to enable them to deliver opportunistic advice to smokers. Smokers contacting the NHS should be asked about smoking and have the NHS smoking cessation services brought to their attention. Those who want to stop should be offered a package of both pharmaceutical aids and behavioural support to meet their particular needs and circumstances. Smokers should have access to a specialist smoking cessation service, and where this is not a desirable option, then other means of support should be discussed (such as telephone and self-help). The National Institute of Clinical Excellence (NICE) has recommended the use of NRT (nicotine replacement therapy) or bupropion (Zyban) for smokers who wish to quit.

Although evidence is currently lacking for most professional groups, other primary health care team professionals should routinely:

- Ask their patients about smoking

- Advise smokers to stop

- Recommend sources of support where appropriate.

A protocol for the dental team to follow is given below (Fig. A1.1). It has been estimated that between 63,000 and 190,000 smokers would stop smoking in a year if all dentists routinely offered smoking cessation advice. Dental professionals offering smoking cessation treatments to patients, including brief

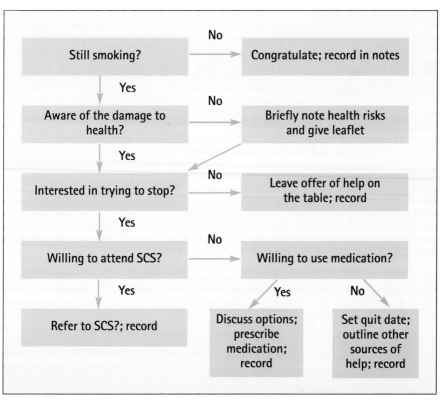

Fig. A1.1. Flowchart for brief advice to smokers. Note: SCS = Smoking Cessation Service. (With thanks to Professor Robert West, Psychology Department, St George's Hospital Medical School, for permission to use this diagram.) (In press.)

interventions, should receive training to equip them with the knowledge and skills necessary to do so effectively.

Key points
• Smokers who wish to give up should be helped by the dental team to do so. *Evidence Base C*

Appendix 2 Guidelines for a healthy diet

The Food Standards Agency (www.food.gov.uk) states that the key to a healthy diet is to eat a variety of foods, which for most people means eating:

- More fruit and vegetables;
- More bread, cereals and potatoes;
- Less fat, sugar and salt.

In more detail, adults should:
- Aim to make up a third of their diet from bread and cereals, choosing wholegrain, wholemeal, brown or 'high fibre' varieties whenever possible.

- Eat at least five portions of fruit and vegetables every day, including fresh, frozen, tinned, dried or juiced. Fruit and vegetables should make up about a third of the food eaten each day.

- Eat a moderate amount of meat, fish and alternatives such as pulses, eggs, nuts and beans, choosing lower fat versions when possible. At least two portions of fish per week should be eaten, one of which should be oily fish.

- Consume less fatty and sugary foods and drinks such as margarine, butter, cream, chocolate and biscuits, and soft drinks, sweets, jam, cakes and ice cream.

- Have milk, cheese, yoghurt, fromage frais and other dairy products in moderate amounts, choosing lower fat versions whenever possible.

- Eat less salty foods. Most adults are eating too much (on average 9g of salt per day – two teaspoonfuls – which should be reduced to less than 6g). Most (about 75%) of the salt in our diets comes from processed foods.

- Drink alcohol only in moderation. Women can drink up to two to three units per day, and men up to three to four units per day, without significant risk to their health. Binge drinking should be avoided. Light-to-moderate drinking of one to two units of alcohol a day has a beneficial protective effect against coronary heart disease for men over 40 and women who have gone through the menopause.

Key points
- Dietary advice for patients given by the dental team should be consistent with general healthy eating guidelines. *Evidence Base C*

Appendix 3 Eruption dates of teeth

Deciduous teeth (months)

Incisors	canines	1st molars	2nd molars
6–8	12–20	12–16	20–30

Permanent teeth (years)

	Lower	Upper
1st Incisor	6–7	7–8
2nd Incisor	7–8	8–9
Canine	9–10	11–12
1st premolar	9–12	9–12
2nd premolar	10–12	10–12
1st Molar	6–7	6–7
2nd Molar	10–12	11–13
3rd molar	17–21	17–21

Appendix 4 First aid for traumatized incisor teeth

It is estimated that about 10% of the population have at least one permanent incisor tooth affected by trauma by the age of 15 years and that many remain untreated. These injuries range from the minor, where the teeth can be restored easily by a dentist, to cases when one or more whole teeth are knocked out. The following advice can be given:

- Professionally made mouthguards should be worn during sporting activities.

- If teeth are fractured, seek immediate dental help and avoid hot or cold liquids and foods.

- If a permanent tooth is knocked out and found, immediate re-implantation can be attempted. The tooth should be held by the crown and contact with the root should be avoided. Any contamination should be removed by rinsing with milk or tap water, but no attempt to clean or disinfect the tooth should be made. The tooth should be supported by biting on a clean folded handkerchief or tissue until seen by a dentist. Re-implantation should not be attempted for deciduous teeth, or if there is any doubt concerning the medical history of the individual.

- If re-implantation is not attempted, the tooth should be placed in a container of saliva or cold milk and taken to a dentist.

- Bleeding should be controlled by biting on a clean handkerchief or tissue for 20 minutes.

- Delay in seeking advice can result in the loss of teeth, which could be saved, or where teeth are knocked out, the movement of adjacent teeth could make the provision of false teeth more difficult.

Appendix 5 Useful evidence-based dentistry websites

- Centre for Evidence-based Dentistry www.ihs.ox.ac.uk/cebd

- Cochrane Oral Health Group www.cochrane.org

- NHS Centre for Reviews and Dissemination, University of York www.nhscrd.york.ac.uk

- National Co-ordinating Centre for Health Technology Assessment, Health Technology Assessment Programme www.ncchta.org

- National Electronic Library for Health – specialist library – Oral Health (dentistry) www.nelh.nhs.uk/oralhealth/dental

- National Institute for Clinical Excellence (NICE) www.nice.org.uk

- Royal College of Surgeons, Faculty of Dental Surgery www.rcseng.ac.uk/dental/fds/clinical_guidelines/

- Scottish Intercollegiate Guidelines Network (SIGN) www.sign.ac

Appendix 6 List of bodies and individuals responding to the consultation

The following bodies and individuals provided comments on this book at the draft stage. Their valuable contributions, representing a broad spectrum of expertise, were gratefully received.

The British Association for the Study of Community Dentistry
The British Association of Dental Nurses
The British Dental Association
The British Dental Health Foundation
The British Dental Hygienists' Association
The Conference of Postgraduate Dental Deans and Directors
The Department of Health
The Faculty of General Dental Practitioners of the Royal College of Surgeons
The Food Standards Agency
The General Dental Council
The National Association of Dentists in Health Authorities and Trusts
The National Oral Health Promotion Group

Ann Davies
Sabrina Fuller
Karen Gonzales
Charlotte Jeavons
Judi McGaffin
Sarah Murray
Mary O'Farrell
Dr T K Ong
Patti Speedy

Appendix 7 List of expert advisers

Prof. A S Blinkhorn	Department of Child Dental Health, University of Manchester
Dr V Clerehugh	Department of Periodontology, University of Leeds
Dr S Creanor	Department of Adult Dental Health, University of Glasgow
Prof. E A M Kidd	GKT Dental Institute, University of London.
Prof. M A Lennon	Department of Oral Health and Development, University of Sheffield
Dr P J Moynihan	Department of Oral Biology and Child Dental Health, University of Newcastle upon Tyne
Prof. D O'Mullane	Department of Oral Health and Development, University of Cork
Prof. A Sheiham	University College Medical School, University of London
Prof. P M Speight	Department of Oral Pathology, University of Sheffield
Prof. E T Treasure	Dental Public Health Unit, University of Cardiff
Dr R G Watts	University College Medical School, University of London

Index

Abrasion 33
'Acid attack' (demineralization episode) 3, 4, 23
Alcohol consumption ix, 64–65
  oral cancer risk 39
Alcoholism 35
Alcopops 35
Anaemia viii, 40, 41, 42
  gingival changes 27
Angular chelitis 40
Antiseptic mouthrinses 28, 32
Aphthous ulceration, major/minor 41
Artificial saliva 42
Artificial sweeteners 22–23
Asian groups, caries prevalence 1
Attendance, dental x
Attrition 33

Benign tumours 37
Betel nut quid 39
Biscuits 9
Breastfeeding 44
Bulimia 35, 36
Bulk sweeteners 22

Cakes 9
Calculus (tartar) 27
  periodontal disease 27
  removal 28
  subgingival/supragingival 27
Candida infection 39, 40, 46, 47
Cardiac defects 15
Caries, dental viii, 1–11, 49

demineralization episodes 3, 5, 7
  with dry mouth (xerostomia) 42
  early childhood 43–44
  effects on teeth 2–3
  health education 51–52, 53
  key points 11
  oral environmental factors 4–7
  prevalence 1
  prevention 7
    diet 9–10
    fissure sealants 11
    fluoride 7–8, 12–18
    plaque control 10, 30
    xylitol-sweetened chewing gum 22
  root caries 47–48
  sugar intake relationship 3, 5, 19, 23, 24
  tooth susceptibility 4
Case-controled studies 56
Cheese 10, 24
Chewing-gum 21
  xylitol-sweetened 22
Children under five 43–45
  key points 45
Chlorhexidine 28, 32
  adverse effects 32
Citric acid 35
Clinical guidelines 57
Clinical studies 56–57
Cochrane Network 57
Cola-type drinks 35
Cold sores (herpes labialis) 41
Confectionery 9
Cross-sectional studies 56